MW01166530

I Trust When Dark My Road: A Lutheran View of Depression

by Todd A. Peperkorn

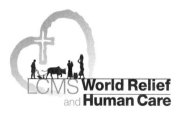

LCMS World Relief and Human Care

Mercy forever.

© 2009 by Todd A. Peperkorn
www.darkmyroad.org

Printed in the United States of America

All rights reserved. No part of this publication may be reproduced, stored in a retrieval system, or transmitted in any form or by any means – for example, electronic, photocopy, recording – without prior written permission of the publisher. The only exception is brief quotations in printed reviews.

Unless otherwise indicated, the Scripture readings used in this book are from The Holy Bible, English Standard Version, Copyright © 2001 by Crossway Bibles, a publishing ministry of Good News Publishers, Wheaton, Illinois. Used by permission. All rights reserved.

Manufactured in the United States of America.

ISBN-13: 978-1-934265-21-5

LCMS World Relief and Human Care
1333 South Kirkwood Road, St. Louis, Missouri 63122-7295
800-248-1930, ext. 1380 • www.lcms.org/worldrelief

To my wife, Kathryn; my pastor, Rev. John M. Berg; and to the people of Messiah Lutheran Church in Kenosha, Wisconsin.

Table of Contents

Foreword

By Rev. Matthew C. Harrison

The anniversary accounts of great pastors and leaders of the church have rarely dealt with the "dark side," the real spiritual struggles and attacks that have often driven pastors and leaders into the abyss of mental illness — clinical depression. I remember reading a document about Synod's second president, Friedrich Wyneken, which stated something like, "Wyneken was always a tireless missionary and pastor, serving courageously for the Lord." Reality is much more nuanced, in fact, much more cruciform. Wyneken wrote to C.F.W. Walther on December 5, 1863 about his lifelong struggle with mental illness and poor health.

> The matter stirred up between us by the devil is finished, dead and buried, I hope to God. But should you, my dear Walther, note something in my demeanor against you, that gives you pause to think — that it may be that the matter still troubles me, do not believe it, but bring the matter openly to me. From the time I was a young man, as far back as I can remember into my earliest childhood, I have suffered horribly from melancholy [depression] and hypochondria, as now in my old age the physical weaknesses all show themselves again, which I already suffered as a child — for instance Asthma. Thus goes it also with my physical nature. How shall I describe it? Hypochondria overcomes me in spite of the fact that I fight and fight against it. I am gripped ever more powerfully by its suffocating arms, so that I am happiest were I had nothing to do with any one, I have to force myself when I have to mingle with people. I am happiest to sit alone in my chair and am consumed in my own stupidity. Then it can happen

that I become very unbearable and my dear brothers must have patience with me, but at the same time they have to correct me quite openly and forcefully. That helps the best, at least for the moment.[1]

Walther was sympathetic. He lived with his own deep struggles with depression, as did his son.[2] Luther knew this struggle too. He faced it both before his understanding of the Gospel, and after. The language he uses in describing the power of the Law breathes of his struggles.

But the chief office or force of the Law is to reveal original sin with all its fruit. It shows us how very low our nature has fallen, how we have become utterly corrupted… In this way, we become terrified, humbled, depressed. We despair and anxiously want help, but see no escape. SA III.II.4

Often, because of physiology and or prolonged stress and other factors too complex to understand, believing the Gospel of free forgiveness does not take away depression. Many go untreated, ashamed, and believing that a "strong faith" would preclude such difficulties, and so the path to wellness is through a restoration of such faith. Not so. "Poor mental health does not necessarily denote poor spiritual health. Too many factors pertain to both to allow for any sure correlation."[3] In fact, in the kingdom of Christ, God values exactly the opposite of what we value. He values weakness,

---

1   Wyneken to Walther, Dec. 5, 1863; Walther Correspondence, Concordia Historical Institute. Translation Matthew Harrison.

2   See Walther's Letter to the German Evangelical *Gesammtgemeinde*, Feb. 3, 1860; Concordia Historical Institute Walther Correspondence, admitting his complete mental and physical breakdown. We would call Walther's condition "clinical depression."

3   Robert Preus, *Clergy Mental Health and the Doctrine of Justification*, Concordia Theological Quarterly, 1984, 48 (2 & 3), 120. Used with permission.

the weakness of the cross.

Most often the "Why do I suffer?" questions are not answered in this life. We do state in faith with the Formula of Concord, that suffering is divinely ordained and purposeful nevertheless:

> God in his purpose has ordained before the time of the world by what crosses and sufferings He would conform every one of his elect to the image of his Son. His cross shall and must work together for good... F.C., S.D. XI.49

Rev. Todd Peperkorn has taken a courageous step in both writing, and allowing this booklet to be published. It is a journey into and through his own deepest struggles. This book will be a profound blessing to many. Pouring forth from the "jar of clay" which is Todd, is a profound stream of mercy, grace, love, and vital experience.

"I will boast all the more of my weaknesses, so that the power of Christ may rest upon me" (2 Cor. 12:9).

Pastor Matthew Harrison
St. Louis
Rogate 2009

Introduction

By Dr. Beverly K. Yahnke

When one's mind and soul journey across the ghastly landscape of clinical depression, the adventure may challenge faith, hope, and life itself.

Far too many well-intentioned Christians are imbued with the conviction that strong people of faith simply don't become depressed. Some have come to believe that by virtue of one's baptism, one ought to be insulated from perils of mind and mood. Others whisper unkindly that those who cast their cares upon the Lord simply wouldn't fall prey to a disease that leaves its victims emotionally desolate, despairing and regarding suicide as a refuge and a comfort — a certain means to stopping relentless pain.

Although Christians are willing to acknowledge that illness and tragedy can befall God's children, many are less charitable about characterizing depression as a legitimate, biologically based illness. Sadly, clinical depression is often misunderstood as a character flaw, a deficit of will or an absence of sufficient faith. Some glance aside, wagging their heads sadly believing that depressed people simply don't choose to "snap out of it" or that they just don't choose to "suck it up" and get on with what it is they've been given to do.

Such myths betray naiveté or ignorance on the part of those who spin them. True clinical depression is not simply a "blue mood" or a bad day at the office from which one rebounds with the dawning of a new day. Depression creeps into every pore of one's life, depriving otherwise nice and normal people of hope, joy, and love. Depression veritably seems to let the helium out of the balloon of life, often insidiously, until souls are left bereft of any capacity or desire to take on even the most fundamental requirements of daily living. Exhaustion and demoralization supplant vibrancy and productivity. The depressed soul withdraws into a cocoon of its own making, isolating oneself from the love and interaction that one desperately needs and desires. In the vacuum of depression there is no energy to do anything, there is no ability to think or to read, there is nothing that invites laughter. Depression must surely be a first cousin to hell on earth, for in the midst of suffering, the soul often feels hopeless and separated from God.

Those of us who have never been afflicted with depression would be absolutely shocked to discover how many of the people in our personal and professional circles have been casualties of mental illness. Conventional estimates of the prevalence of this disease are stunning: one out of every four women will suffer at least one episode of depression during their lifetime; one out of every eight men will experience the illness. The worst news is that nearly two out of three people with depression do not receive the treatment they need either because they have become accustomed to feeling that way, or because their shame about being dysfunction prevents them from seeking care. Still others just keep suffering because at some philosophical level they hate to admit any kind of weakness.

As a result, there are few first-person accounts of the descent into the abyss of depression. For those who have traveled that pathway and who have, by the grace of God, been restored to health, there is often great shame or fear about the prospect that others may learn about their diagnosis and disability. There is often a very legitimate fear that others will misunderstand their illness and judge them in ways that are personally or professionally hurtful or damaging. Very few would regard depression as a life-transforming experience from which one can extract blessing, wisdom, and passion for service.

That is why Rev. Todd Peperkorn's autobiographical account is a gift to us, particularly those of us who are God's blood-bought children. Peperkorn, a Lutheran Church—Missouri Synod pastor, has granted us the privilege of looking deeply into the heart, mind, and soul of a Christian in the clenches of mental illness. We are a bit unnerved to imagine that a Lutheran pastor, called to preach God's Holy Word and to faithfully administer the Sacraments, could possibly suffer such a fate. He challenges all our myths. In his story we see a bright, articulate man serving his church and his parish as God gave Him light. We can detect his zeal for service and love for his family and his people. We watch him enjoying his early successes and we know that God will use this man powerfully. That's why we're shocked to bear witness as Peperkorn describes how he melted away from his parish, his churchly projects, his people, his family, and his friends. We're heartbroken to imagine that any illness could be so catastrophic that it results in God's own servant living in a perpetual fog and having a desire to end his own life.

Peperkorn invites us into the world of a depressed Christian who remains reliant upon God's grace. We walk with him through his early stages of dysfunction until he arrives at a place of professional paralysis, diagnosis, and disability leave from his parish. His journey educates all of us about the realities of clinical depression. He discusses without embarrassment the travails, the treatments, the pharmacological decisions, and the personal struggle that attends the arduous process of healing.

Peperkorn's story also offers us warning and counsel about the way we lead our lives, prompting us to wonder if we, too, might be succumbing to frenetic tangles of productivity and multi-layered obligations. We are invited to re-examine the allocation of our time, re-evaluating whether we are devoting enough precious ticks of the clock to our vocations as spouse, parent, and child — or if we have adopted a plan of embracing our work in lieu of love and life. The text is a particular gift to his brothers, the clergy, as they reflect on their own lives and consider what they have come to believe about mental illness and the spiritual care they offer to souls thus afflicted.

Finally, we see clearly that wearing a stole does not pre-empt depression. In fact, we're led to wonder if clergy, by virtue of all that they are asked to do in service of so many people, might be particularly vulnerable to precisely this form of illness. So, as we greet our pastor at the close of the service this Sunday morning, perhaps we ought to wrap him and his family in prayer, asking that God will equip this man to do all that he is called to do, enfold him in His grace, and sustain him. And we might renew our efforts in every way to support our pastors and their ministry among us.

Preface

In God my faithful God,
I trust when dark my road;
Great woes may overtake me,
Yet He will not forsake me.
My troubles He can alter;
His hand lets nothing falter.[1]

It was Good Friday, but it was not good for me. I was three months into being diagnosed with major clinical depression, and everything was a struggle. For three months I had tried to act like a pastor, even though I was on disability. I preached, taught Bible class, and was "around" far more than the fog in my brain should have let me. So it is that I found myself contemplating my own death on the day of the Lord's death. Contemplating, planning, expecting to die, if not that day, then very soon.

How did I get there? How did I get to the place where I would be considering that darkest of all escapes — suicide — on the day when we commemorate our Lord's death for us all? That is the question this story seeks to answer.

Major depression strikes as many as one in ten people in America[2] — probably more. It is a frightful disease of the mind, turning one inward, sucking out the very marrow of personality, until there is nothing left but darkness. It is a great weight that never lets up, never releases the sufferer from its crushing power. Various studies indicate that the number of pastors who suffer from depression (either diagnosed or undiagnosed) is between 20 and 40 percent.

---

1   *Lutheran Service Book*, "In God, My Faithful God," Stanza 1 (St. Louis, MO: Concordia Publishing House, 2006), 745. Public domain.
2   Mark H. Beers, *The Merck Manual 18th Edition* (Whitehouse Station, NJ: Merck, 2006), 1704.

For many, this is what it means to be a pastor. You suffer, you sacrifice, you can feel the walls closing in and the waters coming up, but you carry on. Why? Because you want to be a faithful pastor.

But no matter how hard you work or pray or exercise or whatever, depression still closes in. You cannot ignore it. Maybe it is because of the stress of the Ministry in 21st century America. Maybe there are triggers in your life — including genetics, or food, or over-stimulation. There are as many opinions as to the cause of depression and anxiety as there are pills to try to cure it. Some things we know. Depression is real, it is devastating, and, for some, it is almost impossible to escape.

So what is the cure? Overcoming depression is not a matter of "cheer up!" or "just have more faith and joy!" or some pious version of "get over it!" I knew the Gospel. I knew all the right answers. I had it all figured out and preached it Sunday after Sunday. But our Lord, in His mercy, chose to crush me, cause me to suffer with Him, so that the faith He gave me in Holy Baptism would be stronger, clearer, and more focused. By traveling down that dark road, I have come to understand what the light of Christ is all about.

Understand that the journey in this book is not the diagnosis of a psychiatrist, the counsel of a psychologist, or the proverbial shoulder of a friend. I write as a pastor, husband, and father. I write because I care deeply about all my brothers in office, as well as all of those to whom they minister. Pastors endure much suffering, often unnecessarily. There are plenty of crosses and suffering that come with the Holy Ministry. There is no reason to take more suffering upon ourselves.

At the same time, I would not give up my sickness today for anything in the world. God has used it to chasten me, change me, make me a better husband and father, and shape me as a better pastor. How is it that such suffering and pain can bring about so much good? Where is God in the darkness and the fog of what we so blithely call "depression" or "melancholy" or even "sadness"?

There is hope, no matter how dark the road. That hope is what this story is all about.

LCMS World Relief and Human Care

12

Chapter One: Building Up to the Fall

No one ever learned anything apart from suffering.
- Malcolm Muggeridge

As a young pastor, I believed I could change the world. I always believed it. I assumed that I was one of the few chosen ones who truly "got it," and that it was my mission to spread the truth to all and sundry, even to most of the other "idiot" pastors out there who didn't get it as well as I clearly did. Perhaps this is a typical sign of youthful exuberance. I'm sure that's true, but it was also a sign of my own arrogance and pride, and in my firmly held belief that I really could do anything. I have the sort of personality that people would call a "connector".[3] I reach out to people, am very comfortable in social situations, and I'm often a leader in whatever groups or settings where I associate. I could do anything.

Everything in my life to that point had borne that out. I was home schooled from 6th through 12th grade. Through the faithful teaching of my father and mother, I learned how to think for myself, do research, take on new projects, and that basically I could go anywhere my mind would take me. Choirs, languages, music, computers, history, and obscure theology books were the building blocks of my high school education. Most of my friends and all of my mentors were older than me. I was more comfortable in a group of adults than with a group of kids my own age. I was used to being alone, playing computer games in the basement, listening to music, going online (very high-tech at the time), and contemplating my future.

---

3   Malcolm Gladwell, *The Tipping Point: How Little Things Can Make a Big Difference* (New York, NY: Little, Brown, and Company, 2000).

Pastors

The pastors of my youth tended to be lively. Two men in particular were instrumental in my own desire to become a pastor. The first was Dale Ness. He and his wife, Hazel, had eight children. He was the pastor at our small church, as well as the sole teacher at our elementary school (20 students in grades K-8). If that wasn't enough, he was also the sole proprietor and worker-bee of Holy Cross Press, a small printing company that produced Sunday school materials, books, and booklets, all on an ancient lightning press that required huge amounts of time to set the plates and make it work. In the eyes of this young boy, Pastor Ness was a hero, a superman among men. As a pastor in my later years, I sought to emulate his endless energy. I didn't realize then that he was pouring himself out on the altar of his own work until there was nothing left.

He was a great pastor, but looking back I can see signs of burnout, stress, and perhaps depression. He put on a cheerful face. He was always singing or teasing and playing with the children. But sometimes he would go through days of melancholy, or the cheerful super-pastor would lose his patience over what seemed to be little things. I don't know if he was ever diagnosed, but much of his behavior could now easily point to clinical depression. He was able to keep going far longer than most people, but eventually he was done.

One Sunday he announced his resignation from the ministry and that he was moving to Idaho with his family. Just like that. There was speculation about burnout, depression, and stress — all of the usual indicators. In three weeks, one of my best friends (Ness's son Peter) and the man I looked up to as a model of what it meant to be a pastor were gone.

The second pastor who influenced me as a young man was Connor Corkran. A feisty Irishman, he was an excellent preacher and a well-trained theologian. He saw in this young confirmand the desire to go beyond memorization into digging, rooting out theological problems, and learning the history of the church. In seventh grade he gave me C.F.W. Walther's *Law and Gospel* as a primer to my theological education.[4] Over the years until he retired, Pastor Corkran gave me all sorts of books to read and digest: Chemnitz, Luther, Pieper, Herman Sasse, whatever he thought might pique my interest. It usually did. Shortly before I went to college he retired. But by then he had filled me with a desire to read and drink in everything I could get my hands on. And with all this knowledge I could do anything.

College

I flew through college with few academic hurdles. The college in the cornfields was a great school; small but challenging, Lutheran but with enough diversity to draw out that feistiness I inherited. I was a leader in everything from choir to yearbook to speech. Greek, Hebrew, and Latin required hard work because I had demanding teachers, but I generally excelled at languages. I dated and participated in large and varied social groups.

The darkness that I would come to know later only flashed in and out from time to time. Sometimes it lasted for days, sometimes weeks. I figured it was just emotions, not enough sleep, girl trouble, or being too busy. I had a friend then whom, I believe in retrospect, suffered from severe clinical depression. I saw him, looked up to him, and observed how he always seemed to pull it off no matter what. It was easy for me to believe, *if he can do it, why can't I?* So I generally did.

One year in particular was full of ups and (mostly) downs. The year is still a blur to me even now. There were lots of late night trips to various food joints under the guise of "homework", but there was little joy. I would wake up for

---

4   C. F. W. Walther, *Proper Distinction Between Law and Gospel* (St. Louis, MO: Concordia Publishing House, 1986). Used with permission.

7:30 a.m. Hebrew and somehow slog myself through the day. I would go back to my room and try to do homework, or keep myself occupied anyway that I could. Anything I could do to distract me from myself was good. Yet through it all I taught myself to put on a good face, appear invulnerable, and never let anyone see the darkness creeping in around me. They probably knew, but I was too blind to see it.

As I left college for seminary, there was no doubt about my future. I would go through seminary easily, focusing either on Hebrew or church history. I would be in the top choir, work on student publications, and after graduation pursue an advanced degree, probably a doctorate. I could do anything.

Seminary

The fog came again not long into my first year at seminary. My girlfriend from college dumped me for someone who was still on campus. I was completely and utterly crushed. I offered to quit my studies for her and rethink my whole future. Fortunately, she still dumped me. Over Christmas break I could barely move or function. Getting out of bed was a victory, and that was often as far as it went. Choir tour (to Florida no less!) was dreary. I didn't care. Yet even then, I was able to mask my true nature.

The fog passed, though, and I was back to taking over the world in no time. I did an inner city vicarage, headed up student publications on campus, and served my regular vicarage in Texas. I married a wonderful woman whom I knew in college. Everything was up with the world.

My fourth year at seminary was messy. It was a difficult time for me as a student and for the seminary community. The seminary president was retiring, and we were seeking another. As student body president, my role as a "connector" was in full swing. There were parties, social events, and committees (even the presidential search committee), while juggling classes, friends, and newly married life. But somehow I managed (in my mind) to hold it all together. Looking back, I can see that depression was beginning to become a way of life. I would expend all of my energy on whatever was in front of me, try to keep all the plates spinning in the air, and every once in a while they would just crash. Each time I would go through "the mood" I would wait it out, perhaps drink more beer, or find other distractions. I didn't know what the cause was. It never occurred to me that there could be some medical explanation.

One thing this did for me was create the idea that real, lasting happiness was for someone else. I would try different remedies to shake off this sinking feeling. It might be alcohol, sarcasm, or popularity, anything that could feed the disappearing ego. What it also did at the time was hone my mask–making ability. I could do all of these things and never let others know the personal struggles I was facing. I never talked about it with my wife, my pastor[5], or any of my close friends. It's as though this fog had enveloped me and I couldn't reach out. Even if I could, I wouldn't know what to say or why.

Seminary Work

For three years after graduation I worked as a seminary admissions counselor. In many respects it was a lot of fun. There was a camaraderie that comes with new beginnings with close friends. There was energy on campus with a new president and new opportunities. The seminary was going

---

5   This is perhaps one of the greatest tragedies of seminary life. As of this writing, neither LCMS seminary has a campus pastor. The home pastors of these men and their families are far away. Faculty members have authority over students, so seeking them out is awkward at best. There simply is no one else. It is no wonder that pastors go out into the field with the idea that they don't need to be cared for themselves. They learn it at seminary.

places: Russia and the whole former Soviet Union, Africa, Asia. We were at the beginning of something big, something significant.

That time was defined, as much as anything, by a way of thinking. It was an attitude of optimism. As the years went on, that attitude of optimism became an unspoken slogan — the invisible uniform everybody wore. If you weren't optimistic and upbeat, then you were not serving the seminary.

I don't say this to fault the seminary, which I love dearly to this day. It is the nature of institutions. Students come, money is given, and things run smoothly — if the appearance of happiness and contentment is what everyone sees. One reason I was good as an admissions counselor was that I knew how to put up a mask and hide behind this façade of optimism. Of course, with any good mask elements of truth make it believable. I *was* optimistic about the seminary. (I still am.) But I was not optimistic about *me*. It became stifling; the stark contrast to my own inner turmoil was too much.

Eventually I could no longer hold up the façade. And when my desire to serve as a parish pastor outweighed my desire to serve the seminary, I accepted a call to Messiah Lutheran Church in Kenosha, Wisconsin.

Messiah

Messiah is a wonderful parish with many loving and caring families. My predecessor lives in the next town over, and we have a good relationship. At the parish level, many things have happened since I've been here. We started a school together with a neighboring parish (Christ Lutheran Academy). There has been an explosion of young families (and thus children) at the church. While the parish has not changed dramatically in size, it has grown spiritually, and has been good to me and my family.

Why is it, then, that after a few short years I began to feel restless, listless? Why was I avoiding my vocation as pastor in pursuit of other enterprises? My compassion and ability to bear others' burdens diminished, and I unconsciously started avoiding unpleasant things I had to do in the parish. I hated the telephone, because it meant I would have to deal with someone in need. I dreaded shut-in calls. Interaction with parishioners became more and more painful. I couldn't handle the stressful situations which every parish has. On top of that, the stress of life with a young family became a burden far out of proportion with reality. I found myself stuck with impossible choices. Do I go to a meeting that will totally deplete me, or go home and struggle to have the energy to play with my children and pretend to enjoy it?

First to go were personal interactions. My open-door policy became a shut-door policy. I hid from people and problems. It seemed like there would be no end to the torture of normal parish life.

What I had most desired had become my cross and my suffering. Sermons started to be recycled or borrowed. The very things that I love most about the Ministry (preaching, conducting the liturgy, teaching) became flat, boring, and one more obligation to carry me down to the depths. After six years, I just couldn't do it anymore. I was going quickly down into the life-draining toilet of depression, and from where I stood there was no way out. I didn't know what was wrong.

So What is Depression?

This is how I have experienced depression, coupled with an unhealthy dose of general anxiety. (More on anxiety later.) Experiences will vary from person to person, as each one's brain acts differently. Depression is difficult to describe. Words like darkness often come to mind; a fog of the brain, walking through thick water, seeing the world as only the faintest of grays, not seeing outside of yourself at all.

To the outsider, depression and other diseases of the mind are a complete mystery. Those who suffer with depression are often viewed as lazy, anti-social, unreliable, high-maintenance, or a problem in some fashion. Because of this misconception, depression, for those who go through it, is something to hide, mask, overlook, or just suffer through in deep silence. You don't talk about it. Though we claim to be enlightened and tolerant, the stigma of depression hits too close to home for many people. It is best not to talk about it at all. Most sufferers don't even know they are sick; depression becomes an undetected cancer of the mind that grows and grows until there is no room for anything else.

We know more about the science of clinical depression now than 10 or 15 years ago, but in many ways our knowledge has remained static. William Styron, in his classic, 1990 autobiographical account of his struggles with depression, *Darkness Visible*, pointed out that depression is chemically induced through the neurotransmitters of the brain.[6] Something goes wrong, and there is a depletion of two chemicals: norepinephrine and serotonin. Accompanying this is an increase in the hormone cortisol. Styron was no doctor, but his basic definition holds up. Even now, almost 20 years later, that clinical definition has hardly changed at all.[7] The psychotherapy versus pharmacology debates of 20 years ago continue to rage, but now we also have alternative medicines, meditation, and many other ways our self-help culture attempts to gain mastery over this disease.

However the inscrutability and the stigma of depression remain as firmly entrenched as 20 years ago. Most suffer in silence, some seek help of one sort or another, but few receive the healing they need in mind, body, and soul.[8]

6   William Styron, *Darkness Visible, a Memoir of Madness* (New York: Random House Publishing, 1990), 47.

7   Mark H. Beers, *The Merck Manual 18th Edition*, (Whitehouse Station, NJ: Merck) 1704ff.

8   Ronald C. Kessler, Patricia Berglund, Olga Demler, Robert Jin, Doreen Koretz, Kathleen R. Merikangas, A. John Rush, Ellen

Depression and Pastors

The above is true for everyone who suffers from depression and/or anxiety in one way or another. For pastors it is worse, or at least has a unique set of problems that are usually overlooked. Why?

New pastors believe they can change the world. They come out of the seminary with a program, a mission to make congregations more Lutheran, more mission-minded, more socially conscious, or whatever the burning issue of the day may be. This program is the special knowledge they have to reveal to their parish. Only they can do it. The people have never heard it (despite the many faithful pastors who went before), and so the new pastor is Josiah discovering the Book of the Law. In his mind he is the messiah to his people, in ways that only he can accomplish. This may sound egotistical, but it is one of the burdens of youth and education. They can be a dangerous combination when they are not tempered by suffering and humility.

Seasoned pastors are comfortable with their role as pastor. They know they can't change the world. All they can do is minister to the people God has entrusted to them. For years they have seen disappointments in the midst of the joys of the ministry. So while the zeal of the new pastor may not be present, the cynicism of the seasoned pastor is no better. Both lead to either a sense of indispensability or doubt of one sort or another.

A part of this mindset is the firm belief that the pastor must always be strong, a rock of certainty to his people who face trials of all shapes and sizes. A pastor must be invulnerable to personal attacks, impervious to matters of his own health and spiritual well-being, and insulated from the lives of his

E. Walters, Philip S. Wang, *"The Epidemiology of Major Depressive Disorder: Results From the National Comorbidity Survey Replication (Ncs-R)"*, Journal of the American Medical Association, 2003, 289 (23).

people, so that he can serve them with what only he can give. This is true for him, and it is also true for his family. The unspoken expectation of having the "perfect" family only increases the pressure of parish life.

It is easy to say that this is a matter of time, age, and patience, but it is true (to some extent). Suffering (*tentatio*) and humility must be learned in the school of experience. The new pastor may theoretically know about them, but his knowledge in the pastoral office is just that: *theory*. The seasoned pastor may have grown used to suffering, but may not fully recognize the relationship between our suffering and the connection it forms with our Lord, the Suffering Servant. If you add into the picture an illness that plays upon the doubts and fears of any pastor, then the pressure is bound to seek release in unhealthy and dangerous ways.

I do not paint these pictures to mock or make fun of young pastors or seasoned pastors. I was that young pastor. The zeal, the sheer joy of going into a new place and a new challenge can be an adrenaline boost like few others. But despite the front that many pastors work so hard to maintain, there is a beating heart under the mask and behind the armor. If that heart, mind, and soul are not cared for there will be much suffering. In the same way, as long as the super-pastor mindset is in place, it is very difficult to be crushed by the hammer of God so that you may serve people not as a demi-god but as an under-shepherd.

This is one of the many ways that depression strikes at the heart of the pastor. I know that this hasn't been a cheery and hopeful picture; but we must understand the reality of suffering that this illness brings upon ordinary people, and its paricular effect on pastors. Don't worry, though. There is hope and healing on the way. We will take the journey together.

Prayer

Lord, with my anxious cares and troubles I come to You, trusting in Your Word and believing in Your promises. You know that I have been greatly upset by the worries, fears, and doubts of the day. You must be my Strength and Refuge if I am to find peace of mind and healing for my body. Uphold me with Your almighty arm.

I am not worthy of Your love and mercy, for I have sinned and often done evil in Your sight. Blot out all my transgressions through Christ's precious blood. Fill my soul with peace. Give me the grace to put all my trust in You. Let Your healing hand rest upon me day after day. Enable me by Your grace to rise above all my suffering to praise You, whose will is wiser than my own. Keep my household and me in Your saving grace, and abide with us all the days of our lives; through Jesus Christ our Lord. Amen.[9]

Questions to Ponder

- Do you see yourself in parts of this picture?

- What factors or people have contributed to making you who you are as a pastor?

- What is it in our lives that make us believe we are invulnerable to suffering and pain?

---

9   *Lutheran Book of Prayer*, Rev. ed. (Saint Louis, MO: Concordia Publishing House, 2005), 229. Used with permission.

Chapter Two: The Place of the Family

The LORD looks down from heaven; he sees all the children of man;
(Ps. 33:13, ESV).

We are not in control of our own bodies, thoughts, emotions, and worldview. Some of these factors have to do with genes, the building blocks from which we came. Each one of us comes from a family, with roots that go back, intertwine, and spring forth in the strangest of places and lives. These other lives intertwine with ours, shape us and form us more than education, work, books, or anything else. If we do not understand how this comes into play, especially when dealing with a disease of the mind, then we are at a great risk of deluding ourselves — believing we are something we're not. Depression certainly runs in families, as do related troubles like anxiety, suicide, and a tendency toward mental illness.[10]

---

10   National Institute of Mental Health, "Depression", Rev. Ed. (Nih Publication No. 08 3561)," 2008,   http://www.nimh.nih.gov/ publicat/depression.cfm.:
"Many years of research have demonstrated that vulnerability to mental illnesses – such as schizophrenia, manic depressive illness, early onset depression, autism and attention deficit hyperactivity disorder – has a genetic component. More recently it has been found that this vulnerability is not due to a single defective gene, but to the joint effects of many genes acting together with nongenetic factors. Despite the daunting complexity, progress is being made.

Researchers are hunting genes because they are likely to be a vital key to deciphering what goes wrong in the brain in mental illness. Detecting multiple genes, each contributing only a small effect, requires large sample sizes and powerful technologies that can associate genetic variations with disease and pinpoint candidate genes ..."

It wasn't until my own illness had sunk in that I began to evaluate myself in light of my family. My wife and children undoubtedly saw how I was changing before I did. My wife knew that I was giving up on things that I used to love. What used to bring me joy now became one more obligation. I looked upon family events as chores to be done in stoic silence, rather than one of the primary vocations in which God has placed me. My wife talked to me about it, but didn't know the cause. I didn't know what to say. Often I would ignore her, or say I would try to do better. No matter how she spoke the words (concern, love, anger, accusation, or just plain bewilderment) it would come across as laying a guilt trip on me. So then a vicious cycle would begin. Not wanting me to feel guilty, she wouldn't talk to me. Or when she did talk to me, I could easily twist it so that she was the one with the problem, not me. How could I explain what I was going through? I didn't understand it myself! Many marriages don't survive depression. I can understand that. It is a testament to her love through Christ that we are still here as a family, and that I am continuing to heal.[11]

If possible, my children (at the time, five and three years old) were even more perceptive. Children have a way of channeling what is going on in their parents. The fact that I couldn't play "chase," or romp around with them, or that I was cross and impatient much the time, all these things shaped them in a way that Kathryn could see, and I was only beginning to perceive. They began to think of me as a bonus part of the family, and not a regular fixture. They would glom on to me for affection so much that I felt smothered, and I would draw back. Any crumb of attention from me was a moment of glee, and any disappointment just reinforced their

---

11   A whole book should be written on the spouses of pastors and how they handle illness, depression, and all its permutations. *The Burden of Sympathy* by David Koch deals with this in more general terms, but the real spiritual challenges remain to be addressed.

unconscious view that I wasn't really there for them. It is clear now, but I didn't see it then. I just knew I couldn't take all that attention and responsibility.

Apart from these general observations about my immediate family, three other family events happened in succession that forced me to look inward even more, and served the illness I didn't know I had. The first was the suicide of my uncle. The second was the death of our unborn child. The third was the death of my mother. These occurred in a six-month period and defined much of what happened afterwards. It wasn't until my wife and I lost a baby that I began to realize what was in front of me and what was slipping away. I also began to look at my family, especially my mother's side, with different eyes. I could see many chapters of my own life story portrayed in impressionist paintings of my relatives – images that reflected my reality, but also leave the imagination to see what is not really there.

Bruce

Everyone has at least one slightly crazy uncle whom they love and admire. In many respects that was my uncle Bruce, my mother's brother. When I was young it was like he was living an adventure novel: scuba diving, water skiing, ski patrol, rock climbing, sports. He owned his own discotheque with the very 70s name of *Suds and Sounds*. My uncle Bruce never lived near us; we didn't see him much. But he was everything a boy *wished* his own father were (at least sometimes). He was exciting. He was active and did wild things just because he could. I loved him then. I love him still.

He was also an alcoholic. In a short time he lost his business, his wife, and everything he owned. He went through a string of wives, jobs, training, houses, and girlfriends over the next 25 years. He moved around some, got into money trouble, and went in and out of rehab programs. No one knew what to do with him, not even my grandfather (Bruce's father), the psychiatrist. But he was family, so everyone kept bailing him out, sobering him up (if possible), and helping him get on his feet. My mother and especially my aunt spent many hours on the phone, making trips, doing all sorts of things to try to save him from himself. He was still sweet, with a mellow and deadpan sense of humor that was infectious. Yet it seemed (at least to me) as though he lived under a curse. No matter what he put his mind to, it seemed to crumble before him.

So it was that in June of 2004 I received a phone call from my father that my uncle Bruce had died suddenly. At the time he lived in a house made of hay bales (!) in Cuba, New Mexico. The trouble was that his parents lived about nine hours away in Colorado. At the time they were in their early 80s and still quite mobile, but we worried about them making a nine-hour trip over mountains to care for their son's remains. I volunteered to fly out and drive them.

My mother, aunt, and cousin met us at the hotel. We drove out, weaving our way up to his house. It was like pulling into some strange sit-com. There was a llama and a three-legged dog. A defrocked priest lived down the road. Various other characters were coming and going. And there was this amazing and bizarre house. He made it out of hay bales, and, in order to have indoor plumbing, built the house around a small RV. It was truly one of a kind. It was a mess. It was his home.

The trip was odd in so many ways. My grandparents weren't Christians, so their views on life and death were quite different from mine. That made the topic of his death a rather uncomfortable subject. Yet that was why we were there: to interpret and understand his death. Through the week my role was to be the solid, stoic one who always thought about the practical things (food, gas, hotels, and sleep). I sought to be strong because everyone else was a basket case. My practice in wearing a mask came into good use once again. Through the viewing, picking up the remains (he was cremated), and the odd service his AA friends held up in the mountains at his home, I was quiet, strong, and practical. No one wanted to know what a Lutheran pastor thought of all of this. It would be too embarrassing to the family. Heaven and hell? Faith in Christ as the only means of salvation? Hope in Baptism alone? I knew it was all true, but they wanted none of it. And I didn't want to make a big fight. I didn't have the energy. So I deferred.

By the end of the week, and by the time I was ready to go home, I was exhausted at so many levels I couldn't count. So many raw emotions. So much pain with no hope. So many people who didn't want to know the truth about Bruce and embrace him, good, bad, and ugly. I had to go home. I felt like I had failed my family by missing the opportunity to offer the Gospel when they were as open towards it as they would ever be. It turned me inward, focused me on my shortcomings and failings. I felt darker than when I left.

Nadia

On Nov. 26, 2004, my wife Kathryn and I lost our baby. Kathryn was 12-weeks pregnant, and the baby had stopped moving. It was over Thanksgiving, so several of Kathryn's family members (including her parents) were around. Kathryn hadn't been feeling well, and we had some suspicions that something was wrong with the baby. So we went to the hospital.

After the ultrasound her gynecologist came in to talk with us. The baby, he said, wasn't alive. It looked like the baby died at about six weeks. We didn't know why (which is typical). The doctor said that at some time the "fetus and other tissue" was going to come out. We could wait for it to come out naturally, or he could perform surgery (dilation and curettage, or D & C) to remove it. I remember the tears and numbness like it just happened yesterday. We didn't know what to do or what to think. No one had told us how to feel.

Kathryn's sister came over and sat with us for a while. Our pastor came over and sang and prayed and cried with us. (He's good at all three.) We decided to have the surgery. It's the same surgery often used for abortion, which made the whole thing all the more dreadful. Plus, a state law said that we couldn't keep the remains for burial. Or at least that's what I think it was. I honestly don't remember. It was all a fog. Our baby went out with all the other hospital leftovers.

By the time we got home, it was late in the day. Kathryn's sister and her family had planned on leaving that day, and decided to keep to their plans. Her parents stayed for a few more days and then went home as well. No one understood the wrenching pain we were in. I don't say this to belittle or criticize anyone. I didn't understand the pain; I could hardly expect others to. They all cared deeply for us, but could not comprehend the depth of our sorrow.

So I put on the mask I knew so well and did services the next day, Bible class and all. I mentioned it in the prayers, and we received a lot of sympathy from the parish. But again, no one really understood, except perhaps those who had gone through it themselves.

That day, our pastor suggested we hold a memorial service. We agreed, and named our baby Nadia.

The memorial service happened the following Wednesday. My father came from Iowa. Everyone else was already home. We had it at our sister church, where our school was in session. I invited members of the congregation by email, and two or three came. Who has memorial services for a miscarriage? Even the term "miscarriage" makes it sounds like you dropped a football, not lost a child. It is dehumanizing and tragic. Profound misunderstanding on everyone's part compounded the numbness and pain. I was mad at my parish, my family, Kathryn's family, God. I was mad at everyone for not taking the death of our daughter more seriously. If a four-year-old child had died, hundreds of people would come, even people the parents don't know. Yet Nadia received no such tribute. It wasn't fair. It seemed as if she didn't count, and that all our talk of being pro-life was just words.

Our pastor did a wonderful job with the memorial Divine Service for Nadia. Despite the small showing of people, it was deeply moving and full of the hope in the Gospel that only a master preacher can give. It consoled us in our hurts and sorrows. He preached on the Visitation, when Mary goes to see Elizabeth (Luke 1:39-56). He shared that God's Word is not bound by our perceptions, that God desires the salvation of all, and that God promises to answer the prayers of fathers and mothers. Then we went to Holy Communion, and Christ was at work comforting us even further.

Yet the heartache and pain were still there, and raw. This didn't fit in a world where I had all the answers. "Why would God do such a horrible thing," I asked myself time and time again. I knew the theological answer, but it didn't matter. Another part of my life became darker.

Mom

Six weeks after Nadia's death my mother, Susan, died at the age of 58. (I was 34 at the time.) For 15 years she had been fighting that vicious disease we call cancer. Hers was melanoma, one of the worst kinds. It had gone into recession, but came back with a vengeance. So her death was not surprising; we knew it was coming. She was at home, and had a sudden brain aneurism as a result of the melanoma. But Mom also had another disease, which I didn't know about at the time.

I had a complicated relationship with my mom. We were very close in many respects, yet we were often at odds with each other (and rarely spoke about it, obviously). We would act as if there were nothing wrong. She didn't say that I shut her out of my life. I didn't feel like she used her illnesses to get what she wanted. Certainly we would never talk about such things. Christians don't act that way, do they?

I am the oldest of four children, 17 years older than my youngest sister. My relationships with my mother and father were different from those of my much younger siblings. I have one sister six years younger than me, so her memories are somewhere in-between. I can remember my mother being active and happy. She was a den mother with Cub Scouts, involved at church, home schooled us all, and was energetic, yet laid-back. I could remember when she would go skiing or play tennis or other sports, which I don't think any of my siblings remember. (I'll hear about it if I'm wrong!)

But about the time I was in seminary, in the early 90s, things changed for her. There was the cancer, to be sure, but it was more than that. My family moved from the St. Louis area to Ames, Iowa, which was very difficult. Although she came to have many wonderful friends in Ames, I don't think she ever felt like it was home. She was a stranger walking amidst friends. So she withdrew. She became quieter and quieter as the years went on. She made fewer visits to family or friends (including me and my family). Her circle of close friends was very tight. During her last few years she rarely left Ames at all. I think her brother Bruce's death was the first reason she interacted with others away from home for several years.

Even when we would visit, it always seemed like she was hiding up in her bedroom. We would drive seven hours to my parents' home, and see her for maybe an hour of the day at most. I resented it. I became angry with her for caring so little about her own children and only grandchildren. Why should we come all that way to visit if she wouldn't leave her room? And she seemed to use the cancer as an excuse to get things her way. If we were in a hurry, she would slow to a crawl. It could take days or even weeks to get a decision out of her for the simplest things. But no one would say anything, because she was sick.

My father, of course, bore the brunt of this. He worked night and day to please her, make her happy, and show her he loved her. But it was never enough. There was always something missing, something more to be done, or some reason not to trust him. It sickened me. For the most part, I blamed her for my father's misery and suffering. Even if he didn't want to speak of it, it hurt him deeply. I believe he began to resent her. A wall of miscommunication went up, and when they needed each other most, Satan was at work prying them apart. Like all relationships, there are always two sides to the story. But I couldn't see my mother's side. My relationship to her had devolved into a polite, distant, yet loving bond, with both of us just waiting for her to die.

When she died I grieved deeply. But I was also relieved that I didn't have to be angry with her anymore. On the plane out I listened to Dvorak's *Requiem Mass*, which gave me a sense of peace, or at least provided focus for my sorrow.

The week of her death was a blur. Family came and went. My own family (and two small children) arrived. Floods of memories and emotions washed over me. It was so fast, so unfocused and messy, that I could barely hold on to reality. But I found a way to escape. I didn't particularly like the pastor (if you're reading this, please accept my sincere apology), and so I bullied my way into preaching my mother's funeral sermon.

If that isn't a sign that something was wrong, I don't know what is. Yet it was the only way I could cope with the situation. It gave me control and focus. I could put on my pastor mask and no one would expect anything else. I could go hide and work on my sermon, and no one would fault me for not spending time with the family. It was perfect. It was sad. It was how I managed things.

The sermon was received well. People were amazed at my maturity and self-control, to be able to preach such a sermon. But for me it was a lie. Every word of the sermon was true, but I did it not to serve or to preach the Gospel. I used that sermon to escape from my own hell. The darkness was into my life, and I was unconsciously fending it off any way I could.

So What?

I've painted these three portraits for a reason. Everyone suffers. It is common to man, and it is a part of who we are, especially as Christians (see Matt. 16:24 and Acts 14:22). I don't think any of these events are particularly unusual, other than their close proximity to each other. But they show something about how depression works into a mind, into a life.

Throughout these events I had all the right answers. I knew what the Scriptures teach about heaven and hell, and that God desires all to be saved and come to the knowledge of the truth (1 Tim. 2:4). I understood God's promises about the prayers of Christians, and that God does not abandon His people in times of trial. He does not want unborn children to be lost, but saved. I realized that even though Nadia hadn't been baptized, she *had* heard God's Word for her short life. And while we could not say with absolute certainty that she is in heaven, we could say with certainty that God is merciful, and that His mercy knows no bounds. I knew the promises of Baptism. I knew that Baptism is powerful because it is the visible Word, and that faith could exist in the most unlikely places and people. I knew all of these things. Yet it didn't matter that I understood them. I could spout off all the right answers, offer comfort and consolation for others, but for myself there was none. I had insulated myself from such things. They were not a part of my world. They were for somebody else, someone who cared, someone who still had feelings.

As I look back on these events, I can see the thread of depression and anxiety running through my family, certainly on my mother's side. My uncle Bruce suffered huge bouts of depression before his death. He largely used America's self-medication: alcohol. That doesn't excuse sinful behavior, of course, but sin always has two sides. We revel in it and are trapped by it. Our Lord came to free us from our sins, and that often means freeing us from ourselves.

In my daughter Nadia's death, I was faced with the horrible realization that I couldn't control my world. I would suffer, hurt, and be in pain for others or myself whether I wanted to or not. It made me very dark, cynical, and angry at God for hating us so much. My reaction was in many respects "normal", yet my mind used those normal reactions to further my illness. The chemicals in my brain weren't working. Depression may be triggered in part by traumatic events in one's life or by a whole host of causes all colliding together.[12] This goes way beyond sadness, grief, or all of the normal responses felt by us sons and daughters of Adam and Eve. Depression triggers a break in the mind so that the usual ways of expressing grief, sorrow, joy, pain, happiness — our healthy human emotions — simply don't work.

In the same way, I had no idea what was really behind my mother's behavior. It wasn't until I went through my own personal hell that I came to realize she suffered from severe depression. She had been on medication for years, and had tried a variety of counselors, doctors, alternative medicine approaches, and a whole array of methods to deal with this sickness of the mind. She was a bathroom smoker, which I didn't know for thirty years. She tried conserving her energy to give one useful, helpful hour to the family each day. I'm not saying she was a saint or the perfect mother. She suffered in silence and bore her burden, for the most part, alone. I don't know if she hid the pain out of embarrassment, to avoid involving her psychiatrist father, or because she believed it was all related to her cancer. But she let few people in, and I don't know if those few choice friends and one daughter truly grasped what she was going through.

My mother's approach and reaction to her depression is

12   David A. Karp, *Speaking of Sadness: Depression, Disconnection, and the Meanings of Illness* (New York: Oxford University Press, USA, 1997), 20.

typical of many. Cases of depression often go undiagnosed or are not treated properly.[13] Many others are under-diagnosed. Sufferers don't receive the care they need. What seems to the outsider like sadness, melancholy, or Seasonal Affective Disorder is in fact far deeper, possibly even deadly.

The Pastor Connection

If this is true for the general population, how much more is it true for pastors? Pastors are taught by word and example to be strong, serve their people and not themselves, and blaze ahead no matter the cost. It is as if the Fifth Commandment doesn't apply (you shall not murder). We pastors don't take care of our own bodies and souls because we believe we have a higher calling. Apparently St. Paul's words have been forgotten by so many of his disciples:

> So to keep me from being too elated by the surpassing greatness of the revelations, a thorn was given me in the flesh, a messenger of Satan to harass me, to keep me from being too elated. Three times I pleaded with the Lord about this, that it should leave me. But he said to me, "My grace is sufficient for you, for my power is made perfect in weakness." Therefore I will boast all the more gladly of my weaknesses, so that the power of Christ may rest upon me. For the sake of Christ, then, I am content with weaknesses, insults, hardships, persecutions, and calamities. For when I am weak, then I am strong (2 Cor. 2:7-10, ESV).

It is not strength, courage, and the model of the Spartans that make the faithful pastor. The faithful pastor is weak for his flock, recognizes his own failings, repents of them, and looks to the Lord for forgiveness — not affirmation for what he believes is good work. Our families shape who we are;

---

13   Depression and Bipolar Support Alliance, "The State of Depression in America: Executive Summary," 1.

David is a prime example in the Scriptures. We cannot escape our roots, nor should we try. If we understand where we came from, it helps put context — flesh and blood — on who we are today. By doing this, the pastor can see his own sufferings and sins more clearly, and Christ will be able to use him all the more as a fellow sufferer with his flock.

Robert Preus, in an insightful essay on the doctrine of justification and mental illness, wrote,

> Pastors who suffer stress and affliction, like any Christian in similar circumstances, may be tempted to look to their faith as a reason for self-esteem and assurance, rather than to the only object of faith, Christ and His pardoning Word. They conclude that failure and inability to cope are due to weak faith or the lack of faith altogether. They are viewing faith as their act rather than as their reception of God's mercy.[14]

Preus holds up an important reality for those of us under the cross. When we are sick, we are always tempted to look inside ourselves for the answers. But the answers never come from within. They come from Christ and His Word.

Throughout much of my life, one Scripture passage has echoed in my ears over and over again: **My flesh and my heart may fail, but God is the strength of my heart and my portion forever** (Ps. 73:26, ESV). Only the reality that God Himself sustains me, no matter what may come, can pierce the heart of a troubled soul. As a pastor, I am often tempted to mask myself, pretend to be something I'm not, in order to fulfill some fantasy about what people want in a pastor. The reality is that it's not about me. This applies to pastors and to anyone. God alone is our strength. May it ever be so.

---

14   Robert D. Preus, "Clergy Mental Health and the Doctrine of Justification," *Concordia Theological Quarterly* 1984, 48, (2 & 3), 120. Used with permission.

Prayer

O God, you resist the proud and give grace to the humble. Grant us true humility after the likeness of Your only Son that we may never be arrogant and prideful and thus provoke Your wrath but in all lowliness be made partakers of the gifts of your grace; through Jesus Christ, our Lord. Amen.[15]

Questions to Ponder

- Where does your family fit into your worldview?

- Can you learn anything about yourself from understanding the strengths and failings of your own family?

- If so, how does that affect your approach to the Holy Ministry?

---

15 *Lutheran Service Book* (St. Louis, MO: Concordia Publishing House, 2006). 312. Used with permission.

Chapter Three: The Early Signs That Things Were Wrong

Entrust your days and burdens
To God's most loving hand;
He cares for you while ruling
The sky, the sea, the land.
For he who guides the tempest
Along their thunderous ways
Will find for you a pathway
And guide you all your days.[16]

I began to realize things weren't right with me when I began missing home and family events on purpose. I would create excuses, claim a need to work, or (subconsciously) develop illnesses so that I didn't have to interact as much with my family. I kept so busy with projects, things that simply couldn't wait, that I didn't have time for my own wife and children. It was easier to work on a project (especially on the computer) than to interact with anyone.

In retrospect I can see what was going on, at least in part. Social withdrawal is a key mark of major depressive disorder.[17] It is hard to understand, especially for the spouse, friend, or relative. From the outside it may appear that the depressed person is angry with them or has given up on their relationship. The reality is that the depressed person may not even be aware of what's happening.

I fought this in several ways. In the spring of 2004 my wife and I trained for a marathon. Typical of my personality, if I'm going to do something it has to be the most impressive

---

16   *Lutheran Service Book*, "Entrust Your Days and Burdens," Text, (sts 1.) (St. Louis, MO: Concordia Publishing House, 1982), LSB 754. Used with permission.
17   Mark H. Beers, *The Merck Manual 18th Edition* (Whitehouse Station, NJ: Merck, 2006), 1705.

activity, with the best equipment, reaching as far as I can possibly go. The marathon is a perfect example of that excess for me. We trained. I lost weight. I ran and ran and ran and ran. I knew I wasn't cross-training like I should. Considering my weight, my age, and my lack of history with running, I knew that I was over-training and lacked the kind of cross-training necessary to do it well and actually enjoy it. So it was no surprise that my knee broke down on a twenty-mile run. I couldn't run for a while. I had to see a doctor. My wife went on alone. I received lots of sympathy, but also lots of time to myself — and lots of reasons not to do things with the kids and others.

Several months later, we actually did run a marathon together. I trained a little more carefully, spent more money on shoes and other running gizmos, and, despite the risks, we went ahead with the run. My knee gave out at about mile 13, and we had to walk three miles before we could start running for three minutes at a time. Some how we finished, after I got taped up and pumped full of Ibuprofen at an aid station. This time I got the accomplishment, the positive feeling of actually *doing* something, *and* I got to use an injury to disengage more. What could be better?

At the time I used either work or physical problems (both real and exaggerated) to disengage, to run away from the human interaction that was becoming more and more difficult to maintain. The things I was avoiding started to pile up. Vacations became torture. Even short outings were something to dread, not look forward to and enjoy. Any interaction — especially confrontation — drained me so that there was nothing left. The work of being a pastor at a church with a young school, all of the extra-curricular distractions (another chapter), and my family together sucked out everything I had. Responsibilities slipped in one area, then another. I couldn't keep all of the plates spinning, and began dropping things in a frantic attempt to stay in control and keep my sanity. I chose what was most important to me, and those choices hurt a lot of people.

The following is an entry from my blog-journal in the middle of my year of disability and recuperation:

The Fireworks

I'm sitting at home tonight alone. My family is off doing the annual fireworks display thing downtown. I can't go. The noise. The people. The clutter. The questions from my children. I just can't take it. It would wear me down. My brain would overload. I would get nervous and jittery, like too much caffeine. Then I would start to shut down. I would turn into a zombie. Staring into space, praying for the noise to stop.

It's not that I don't like fireworks. Okay, truth be told, I've never been a huge fan of fireworks. But we've always gone to the fireworks. It's what you do on the 4th. Duh. But not this year for me. I just couldn't take it.

This is, of course, simply one of many examples of things I have missed because of my illnesses. Between depression and anxiety (two illnesses that often go hand in hand), I have missed a lot over the years. Graduations. Confirmations. Birthdays. Recitals. Even little things like walks to the park, extended family events. The list could go on and on.

And this is just family, of course. If we started to talk about church, I'm not even sure where to begin. For me, the most obvious and painful is preaching and teaching. I love preaching and teaching. It's why I became a pastor. Yet my mind doesn't allow me to function well enough right now to do it. I used to be just numb to this. Now I'm more anxious to get back into things. I'm sure my counselor would tell me this is a good sign.

But whether we're talking about family or church or other parts of life, the reality is that depression and anxiety just plain change things. You can't do these things. At least for a time.[18]

The feeling that your life is slipping away is maddening. It doesn't necessarily create sadness, though it can make you sad, angry, frustrated, anxious, out of control, and a host of other things. But usually depression leads to feelings like guilt, shame, relief (which leads to more guilt), a numb nothingness, and despair. How did I deal with this? How do we find our way out of this jumbled mix of medical conditions that Satan uses to drive us to despair, devoid of all hope? Here are a few thoughts:

- **Guilt.** I believe I should be able to do all the things I normally do. If I had a broken leg, would I feel guilty for not being able to walk? Maybe, but it would be pretty silly. Why is this different? Guilt is about sin, and there is forgiveness in the blood of Christ. But this is not really guilt. Satan wants me to believe I am guilty of some wrongdoing so he can take me down his dark road.

- **Shame.** I'm embarrassed to be so weak and incapable. (This, by the way, can be the backside of pride.) The concept of weakness and suffering does not come easily to pastors, especially younger pastors. I may know all the right answers about suffering, but it is different when I am in the middle of it.

- **Relief.** I know I can't do these things, so it is liberating to be free of them at least for a time. A period of rest (sabbatical) is a good thing. But we are so programmed to go, go, go until we drop, that this relief is often fleeting. Then guilt returns. It is not a sin to be sick. It is not a sin to seek relief when you need it. Our Lord Himself often went into retreat, to

---

18   http://www.darkmyroad.org/?p=8, July 4, 2006.

have time alone to pray, meditate on the Word of His Father, and rest. He Who is our Sabbath rest invites us to rest. Yet somehow pastors have bought this crazy notion that rest is for the weak, and weakness is bad. It is not so.

- **Creepy despair.** Will I ever be able to do the things I enjoy again? Or have I given them up for good? Will I ever be the person I once was, or will I remain this shadow of my former self? Despair is more theological than medical. See the Sixth Petition of the Lord's Prayer. Satan causes despair by using the events in our lives to lead us away from where our confidence lies (Christ and His gifts) and turn us toward ourselves or something or someone else for hope. Despair is creepy, and it creeps into the most unsuspecting places. Giving up things in your life, intentionally or unintentionally, leads to guilt, and guilt leads either to repentance and forgiveness, or despair.

- **Hope.** Temporary relief from the responsibilities of life is a gift, but it can be hard to see. Hope is elusive, like relief. But it will come, as sure as the morning. Even when you don't feel it, when you can't see it, know that it is there. For most who suffer from depression, there is a profound period of hopelessness. Days, weeks, even years are lost to the feeling that nothing will ever be the same again, that one will never be rid of this weight. Hope is persistent, though, because it is based on the certain promises of Jesus Christ, who suffered utter hopelessness on the cross for our sake. ("My God, my God, why have you forsaken me?" Ps. 22:1) Even in our darkest moments, Christ will not abandon us.

I still go through these feelings every day, even now — long after my darkest moments. Some days all of them hit me.

The hope took months to come, and only after being fed by the Word of God, which I had denied myself for so long. In the midst of the horror of depression, even hearing the Word of God, praying, and receiving His gifts can be painful.

How can hearing God's Word be painful? For the pastor, hearing God's Word from someone else can translate into questions. "Why can't I do that anymore? What is *wrong* with me?" My pastor and I had a conversation about this partway through my year of disability. I found that when I went to church I couldn't participate. All I could do was sit and stand when I was told. I had to re-learn how to listen, how to receive. Sometimes all you can do is receive. This may sound like a failure on our part, but it is a profound gift from God to understand that worship and faith are reception. Our confessions put it this way:

> Thus the worship and divine service of the Gospel is to receive from God gifts; on the contrary, the worship of the Law is to offer and present our gifts to God ...This passage, too, brings the greatest consolation, as the chief worship of the Gospel is to wish to receive remission of sins, grace, and righteousness. Of this worship Christ says, John 6, 40: This is the will of Him that sent Me, that every one which seeth the Son, and belieiveth on Him, may have everlasting life.[19]

In the midst of depression, and when attacked by despair, it is a great comfort to know that God does not expect you to *do* anything. I love singing, leading the liturgy, preaching, and giving out His Sacraments. But it took the numbness of my mind to help me remember that worship is receiving, not giving. Only in Christ do we find relief, and we only find Christ through His gifts freely given *to* us.

19   Paul Timothy McCain, (ed.), *Concordia: The Lutheran Confessions – A Reader's Edition of the Book of Concord*, 2nd ed. (St. Louis, MO: Concordia Publishing House, 2007), AP III paragraph 189. Used with permission.

This concept of relief also took time to sink in for me. It is so often contrary to our nature as pastors. I wonder if that has always been the case, or if this trial is unique to our age. I know many pastors who never take even one day off. Others take a "day off" to do all the cleaning up and other work around the church. Pastors, in a desire to be faithful, can very easily rob God's flock of her vocation of caring for her shepherds and God's house.

I remember years ago having a conversation with a dear parish member who was dying of cancer. He was the sort who was always there, willing to help, making things (woodworking in his case), doing anything in his power for the sake of his church. Everyone loved him. He came to see me not long after finding out about his illness. He had no fear of whether he would go to heaven; his faith was sure, as only Christ can make it. Rather, his greatest fear was of being a burden to his children and grandchildren. They were all so busy and had so many things going on in their lives, how could they have time for him? In one of those pastoral (Spirit) flashes that occur every so often I told him, "Sometimes, Merle, the greatest way that you can help another person is to let them help you. Your family loves you deeply. You've raised them, taken care of them, and even now you want to take care of them. The best way you can take care of them now is by letting them have the joy of taking care of you."

Pastor, heal thyself. Or more accurately: Pastor, allow the Spirit's words from your mouth to work also on you.

Prayer

I want some answers
Lord
clear directions
final solutions
but without
too much anxiety

or pain
on my part
but my demands
are wrong
Instead awaken me
to the biblical truth
that *discovery*
may only come
through *crisis*
distress
grief
even agony
and that
as I share in
your sufferings
and those of others
I also receive
your comfort[20]

Questions to Ponder

- How have you sought to escape from the pressures of your family and your parish? Have you been honest with yourself and others regarding what you are doing and why?

- Why is it that pastors are so afraid to admit weakness, seek relief, and ask for the help of others?

- How does the example of our Lord seeking solace give you comfort?

---

20   Donald L Deffner, *Prayers for People Under Pressure* (Milwaukee, WI: Northwestern Publishing House, 1992), 35. Reprinted with permission.

Chapter Four: The Pill That Marked Me

Bow down Your gracious ear to me
And hear my cry, my prayer, my plea;
Make haste for my protection,
    For woes and fear
        Surround me here.
Help me in my affliction.[21]

At Christmas time I found myself overwhelmed. I'm not talking about the position that is tragically typical of pastors around Christmas. I was non-functional. Advent was torture. I gave up making calls. Normal tasks became like wading through molasses. I couldn't plan services. I could barely write sermons, if at all. More and more I borrowed sermons. Events like a Christmas party or caroling with the choir filled me with dread.

This was very odd for me. I am a social person by nature, a "connector" as I said near the beginning. Parties, social gatherings, speaking before large groups, preaching, teaching — these things came quite naturally to me. That I dreaded these very things that had been part and parcel of my character for so long was a sign something was not right. What was wrong? Even at that point I didn't know, and would not have guessed.

The other telltale sign was that I couldn't see past the day in front of me. Even more, I began to forget things. Whole blocks of time began to simply disappear. I can remember what was going on then better *now* than when I was in the middle of it. I couldn't remember what was happening before, would forget even the most mundane things, and couldn't see much more than two days ahead, if that. Most doctors would tell you

---

21 *Lutheran Service Book*, "I Trust, O Lord, Your Holy Name," Stanza 2 (St. Louis, MO: Concordia Publishing House, 2006), 734. Public domain.

that was textbook depressive behavior, but I couldn't see it.

I masked it. I masked it with back pain (very real), headaches, and being tired. I would mask it with any excuse. If only I could get more sleep, get my back to heal, or any of a hundred other things, then surely I would feel better. Then I would be back to my old self, and things would be normal again.

It was a lie I told myself in order to avoid seeking real help. Yet it seemed like the only way I could cope with the pain, the inner demons that were driving me to despair.

The trip to my wife's parents was equally difficult, if not more so. We drove the ten hours to her parents, where all of the siblings gathered into one house, along with mom and pop. There must have been 20 people in the house, ranging from two to 75 or so. It is the sort of ordered chaos that should only happen in families; otherwise there would be serious Fifth Commandment issues. But it's worked for years so we were at it again, the triennial pilgrimage home.

For me it was painful beyond measure. My back was seriously hurting, but even more, this overwhelming sense of dread and creeping darkness was ever present. I couldn't stand to be with other people (even my own wife and kids), and I couldn't stand to be alone. I wanted very much to be a part of what was happening, but it was like there was an invisible wall separating me from them. I couldn't get through. I could only see them, and know that I was not a part of it.

In retrospect, I am amazed at my own blindness. How could I not see what was happening to me? My wife knew something was wrong, but we had no way of knowing or understanding what it was. When physical problems and mental anguish are mixed, it is very difficult to pull them apart for diagnosis, moreso if it is happening to you. You keep hoping once this or that pain goes away, the mind will settle back down to normal. Furthermore, depression manifests itself in men differently than in women.[22] Some men exhibit depression by being irritable, angry, or profoundly discouraged. It can easily be mistaken for just having a bad day or week. In my case, we didn't recognize it for months.

One of the things many people don't realize is that depression has real, physical consequences.[23] With those little neurotransmitters not working right, your brain is desperate to tell your body that something is wrong. This can be made manifested in obvious things like mood swings. It can create a lack of libido. Headaches, backaches, and the physical manifestations of stress also accompany depression. In fact, stress is one of the chief triggers of depression in America.[24] How can the depressed person determine the root cause of these symptoms?

By the time our family trip finally ended, mental and physical anguish had turned me into a great big mess. I knew then that more was at stake than my evident physical ailments. It was not just my back; there was something wrong with my mind.

The Doctor

Upon returning home I went to my family doctor and explained more or less what was going on. He suggested that I go on welbutrin, a common anti-depressant and one of two major types.[25] I told him I'd think about it. He told me welbutrin would help with depressive problems as well as obsessive-compulsive behavior, and would assist in weight loss.

It made sense. I knew this might be a step in the right direction, but first I wanted to speak with someone I really trusted.

---

22   Strock, *National Institute of Mental Health*, "Depression," http://www.nimh.nih.gov/publicat/depression.cfm (1994).

23   *Ibid.*

24   *Ibid.*

25   *Ibid.*

The Point of Fear and the Voice of Reason

Several steps on this journey cause me pain even now when I recall how hard they were. They struck at the core of my super-pastor image, which I had fought so hard and long to uphold. The first was a simple phone call. I knew a psychologist about 45 minutes away, to whom I had referred parishioners over the years. We had worked on various church projects together, so we were acquainted but not close. She was the obvious person for me to call.

That call was one of the most difficult things I've ever done in my life. It seemed like an admission of failure. It proved that I was all washed up as a parish pastor, and that my pride had led me so high that everything was about to come crashing down. It's amazing how much thought we can invest in one simple act, isn't it? Yet there it was. I waited a week, almost two, but the pain became unbearable. The pain of *not* seeking help was worse than the fear *of* seeking help. I finally called. We had a short conversation, and she invited me to come in for a no-strings-attached evaluation. The ice had been broken, so I could enter the cold waters that led I knew not where.

My first visit with the psychologist/counselor soon arrived. I was afraid. I brought my pastor along for moral support. She did a number of evaluations and determined that I was suffering from major clinical depression. I did not know the depth of it, but there was some relief in knowing, "I'm not crazy! I have a mental illness!" We discussed medication options, and she encouraged me (in a non-directional lead-down-the-path way common among therapists) to seek medical treatment in addition to seeing her. I told her my doctor had recommended welbutrin. She said it was a good, common anti-depressant with a good history, and had been used by many people with much success.

The Pill That Set Me Apart

When I got home, I called the doctor and ordered a prescription for the medication. After I picked it up from the pharmacy, it sat on the shelf. I don't remember how long it sat there; maybe a week. What I do remember is looking at those pills and seeing them as a mark of failure which I could never overcome, from which I would never recover. If I started taking these pills I would be damaged goods. My whole future as a pastor seemed wrapped up in this tiny pill. I knew I needed it (or something), but I was afraid, deeply afraid of taking this trip into the cold dark waters.

Why was I so afraid? It was just a pill. I've taken lots of pills in my lifetime, but this one was different. It seemed as though this pill would change my identity. Dr. David Karp speaks about this in his masterful work, *Speaking of Sadness: Depression, Disconnection, and the Meanings of Illness.*[26] In this book, Dr. Karp, a sociologist and fellow sufferer of depression, did a case study of 50 individuals from all walks of life who had suffered or were suffering from depression in various stages. One of the issues that Karp identifies is the combination of illness and identity (chapter 3). Karp describes how, at different times in history, various things have been labeled as illness and others as normalcy.[27] The terms, to some extent, are social constructions. In the 1960s, for example, it was quite popular among social scientists to view depression as an arbitrary construction and not an illness at all. It was a way of casting "different" people outside of the mainstream, into the murky realm of the mentally ill. Meanwhile, leaders in the Soviet Union were labeling "insane" everyone who disagreed with the state, and putting them away like so many dogs.

To my knowledge, Karp is not a Christian, so his views on

26 David A. Karp, *Speaking of Sadness: Depression, Disconnection, and the Meanings of Illness* (New York: Oxford University Press, 1997).

27 *Ibid*, 54-55.

many things will differ from ours. However, he understands how an illness can become part of one's identity. A host of words make this connection: paralytic, diabetic, quadriplegic, and so on. Yet many major diseases do not take on this identity factor, such as heart disease, cancer (to some extent), and Lou Gehrig's disease.

The Pill and the Pastor

Why only some diseases cast an identity is beyond my understanding. I can, however, talk about identity and why taking a pill or seeing a psychologist may be so difficult for a pastor. While pastors wear many hats (son, husband, father, citizen, etc.), there is a very real sense that the identity of pastor supersedes all others, whether it should or not. Maybe it is our high view of ordination and the divine call. Maybe it is just drilled into us as we become pastors. I don't know. But it is certainly true that pastors take quite seriously this identity as one who speaks in the stead of Christ.

Now this is good, because the pastoral office is a high and holy calling. However, pastors may end up with such a skewed view of themselves that their view of our Lord becomes messed up in the process. If a pastor believes that he can never show weakness, that he must always be strong for his people, and that the only way to serve them is by being impervious to illness or problems, then the thought of taking a pill which might change your identity (even in your own mind) is a huge step. It means becoming someone else. It means rethinking your view of the pastoral office. It may mean asking whether you can be a pastor at all.

There are many fine men out there who have been lost to the pastoral office because of depression and how they and their congregation handled it. So it should come as no surprise that taking this pill became a mark, a turning point, in how I saw myself and how I would address this newly diagnosed disease called depression. It was a step, but it was painful.

As I think back on that step, it is obvious that I could never have taken it alone. My wife, pastor, counselor, and the few trusted friends in whom I had confided all played major roles in my healing. Just as God provides spiritual relief through His Word, He provides physical relief through people. *Give us this day our daily bread* means more than the food on the table. It means *everything* we need to support this body and life. Thank God that He puts into our paths people who may be Good Samaritans to us, and lift us up when we have been left for dead.

Prayer

Lord, you are the great Physician of body and soul. You alone can calm the fears of your sick children. Help me to recognize my own needs, and to seek the help that only comes by your mercy, so that I may be healed, restored, and made anew in your image; through Jesus Christ, our Lord. Amen.

Questions to Ponder

- Have you ever had an identifying event that shaped your whole life? What was it?

- What are you most afraid of as a pastor?

- Where do things like pills or psychotherapy fit into our theology? Are they strictly left-hand kingdom (Law), or can they used by God's right hand (Gospel)?

Chapter Five: Anxiety

Anxiety is a thin stream of fear trickling through the mind.
If encouraged, it cuts a channel into which all
other thoughts are drained.
-Arthur Somers Roche

Pill number one was a disaster. By the time I got around to taking it, I had to leave for a week-long trip — the annual seminary pilgrimage known as symposia. Very shortly after I started taking welbutrin I got ill: nausea, dry mouth, severe anxiousness, a flu-like headache. Now I was depressed, sick, and crabby to be away from home during all of this. I barely went to any lectures, and the fellowship of pastors (often including beer) left me empty and cold. All I wanted to do was leave. I had made this hard choice to start taking the medication, and now even the medicine was messing me up!

By the time I got home I could barely move. I was empty, tired, sick from the medication, and feeling no closer to any kind of solution. My doctor told me that it sometimes takes a week or two for the medication to settle into your system. Give it a little more time, he said, and it will get better.

It didn't; it got worse. The flu-like headaches became a little easier to bear, but the anxiety was getting worse and worse.

Anxiety

Anxiety is hard to pin down. It often goes hand in hand with depression. Many people hear the word anxiety and think of an emotional state of mind, much like the common view of depression. The biblical band-aid often applied to anxiety is taken from St. Paul's letter to the Philippians 4:

Rejoice in the Lord always; again I will say, Rejoice. Let your reasonableness be known to everyone. The Lord is at hand; do not be anxious about anything, but in everything by prayer and supplication with thanksgiving let your requests be made known to God. And the peace of God, which surpasses all understanding, will guard your hearts and your minds in Christ Jesus (Phil. 4:4-7, ESV).

Taken out of context or in the wrong sense, this verse can easily be interpreted as, "Don't worry, be happy. If you do this, God will take care of you." It's a nice law approach, meant to be very comforting. However, we need to distinguish between a theological world-view (not trusting God to take care of the future in Christ), and the very real medical issues of depression and anxiety.

I have come to think of anxiety as a phobia. People can be afraid of tight places (claustrophobia), spiders (arachnophobia), or a host of other things. Such a fear is irrational. It grips you so that you cannot get away, while convincing you that if you stay in the situation something really bad will happen. The sufferer of a severe phobia may be driven to hurt him- or herself or others in order to escape the fear.

Welcome to the anxiety half of depression.

Anxiety Magnified

I had experienced anxiety before, but somehow that drug magnified my sense of anxiety, nervousness, and unease with the world around me. I began to fear crowds, stress, responsibility, my children, noise — virtually any kind of stimulation became a huge burden and scared me near to death. I spoke with my counselor, tried to give it another week or two, and then things really fell apart.

One day (I think it was a Friday) I could feel my heart racing. I wasn't doing anything. I had given up caffeine by then, so there was no real explanation other than the drug. But what was my conclusion? I thought I was having a heart attack. *I'm 35 years old and I'm having a massive heart attack!*

My wife couldn't calm me down. Nothing seemed to work. After two or three hours of this torture, I finally called my doctor and asked if I could come in.

The doctor's office got me right in, had me put on one of those crazy hospital gowns, and shaved some of the hair off my chest in order to give me an EKG. After a great deal of attention in a short amount of time, they determined that my heart was fine and that it was all in my head. (They said it more politely than that.) The doctor took me off welbutrin and put me on a common anti-anxiety medication called Xanax. That got me through the weekend.

Shortly thereafter I went to a competent psychiatrist, who proscribed a different anti-depressant (sertaline/Zoloft), a different anti-anxiety medication (clonapam), and a sleeping medication (trazedone). After mixing the cocktail different ways over the next 10 months, eventually we hit on the right combination. It even included welbutrin again when the sertraline alone wasn't doing it.

This experience is fairly common when addressing depression and anxiety. Each body is different, and there are dozens of medications for various aspects of depression. It can take time to find the right combination, sometimes a long time. And after a while, one combination might no longer work, and a new balance must be found. Medication can be expensive, insurance companies will try to dictate what to prescribe, and the patient quickly gets sick of the whole process.

This scenario may be true of any injury or medication, but with depression and anxiety, it compounds the problem. When you're in the middle of it you can't think clearly enough to make intelligent decisions. You have invested so much energy into the decision to take the pill(s) that the thought of changing or having to fight to keep them weighs much heavier than it would otherwise. In the end, it is the disease that makes the treatment process so difficult and painful.

A Team Effort

This is why it is so important to have a team of people who will help you through all the decisions. You can't make them alone. Your spouse, a competent counselor or psychiatrist, your pastor — all can serve as God's instruments to bring hope and healing. He may use them in different ways and at different times, but He will use them all. Our Lord wants you to be healed at the proper time. He does not wish for you to suffer needlessly, but wants you to be whole and complete in Him.

As pastors we are often tempted to think of ourselves as the solution to every problem. It goes with the super-pastor identity. A good doctor knows when to refer his patients to a specialist. A good pastor needs to know when part of the problem is not within his realm to heal.

Prayer

Dear Lord, I know that you own even more and have more in storage, than you have given away. In you I shall not want. If need be, the heavens indeed would pour down a supply for our need. You will never fail me. You make me rich. If I have you, I have all I want. Amen.[28]

Questions to Ponder

- What is the difference between being anxious, as mentioned in the Scriptures, and anxiety as a medical phenomenon?

- Why don't pious remedies and platitudes cure anxiety?

- What does ease the pain and stress of anxiety?

28 Martin Luther, *Luther's Prayers* (Minneapolis, MN: Augsburg Fortress Press, 1994), 100. Reproduced with special permission.

Chapter Six: So Is it real?

I waited patiently for the LORD; he inclined to me and heard my cry.
He drew me up from the pit of destruction, out of the miry bog, and set my feet upon a rock, making my steps secure.
(Ps. 40:1-2, ESV).

Is depression real? We're a long way into this little book and have yet to answer this basic question. Many people claim that depression is not a legitimate medical illness but a social construction.[29] Others have gone so far as to say that depression is the result of supply and demand: Pharmaceutical companies have created these drugs, and their marketing departments and our consumerist society give depression more life than it had in decades past.[30]

Nor is the church immune to such views. Seventy-six years ago a Lutheran pastor had this to say about depression:

But if we cling to the promises of God, we shall yet praise Him for the help which He has given us in the days of adversity. Therefore our souls should not be cast down. We Christians have no right to be depressed or blue.[31]

The book was reprinted at least four times, and continued

---

29   Allan V. Horwitz, *Creating Mental Illness (Culture Trails)* (Chicago: University of Chicago Press, 2003). See also A.B. Curtiss, *Depression is a Choice: Winning the Battle Without Drugs* (New York: Hyperion, 2001), and A.B. Curtiss, *Brainswitch Out of Depression: Break the Cycle of Despair* (Escondido, CA: Oldcastle Publishing, 2006).

30   Bret Stephens, "The Great Depression: Richest Country, Saddest People – Any Coincidence?," *The Wall Street Journal* (March 9, 2007).

31   Alfred Doerffler, *The Burden Made Light* (St. Louis, MO: Concordia Publishing House, 1937), 21. Public domain.

to be used through the 1980s. This was before the age of clinical diagnosis of depression. However, our church has not progressed far since 1931. In *Pastoral Pitfalls in the Church* (1997), Kurt Brink equates depression with sadness, frustration, and a desire to quit the ministry, and sees it as fundamentally (solely) a theological problem — possibly a sin.[32] This view, common in many parts of our society, stands out as cruel in the church. Most congregations have a poor record of serving pastors who suffer from depression or other mental illnesses. I say this not to criticize my church, but to point out that no one is immune from the views of the world and the prevailing winds of science. Although many have tried, and continue to try to improve the situation in our church, relief is not arriving quickly. The rate of attrition in pastors is terrible, and there is no evidence at this point of it turning around. When pastors become ill, or their future is uncertain, the possibility is very real of their leaving the ministry and never coming back.

When the Disease Hits the Road

This is the context in which I lived as I considered my future as a pastor. I was on medication, but was continuing downhill fast. My level of functionality was getting worse by the day or even the hour. I resigned or took an extended leave of absence from all non-parish work with which I was involved. It was not enough. The church, our school, and my family were the three things requiring the most energy. I couldn't simply give up on my family, nor would I consider it. Something had to give.

I spoke to our congregational president and head elder about my health situation shortly after starting to take medication. We told the rest of the elders soon thereafter. The congregational leaders were aware that I was going through

---

32   Kurt Brink, *Overcoming Pastoral Pitfalls* (St. Louis, MO: Concordia Publishing House, 2003), 17.

significant medical problems, and were supportive, inspite of not understanding. I don't blame them. I didn't understand it myself, and could hardly expect them to.

Whom Do You Tell?

This raises a serious question facing pastors that suffer from depression. Whom do I tell? Your wife knows early on. Do I tell members of my parish? Who else? *Great,* I thought to myself, *the more decisions I have to make, the less I am able to make them.*

This is a very real dilemma for pastors. Part of the problem is pride. I don't want my people to know that I'm sick with a mental illness. Some of the fear is quite legitimate. I have seen pastors kicked out of parishes for "being lazy," resigning their call and going on candidate status, never to return. I've seen pastors refuse to tell anyone, and suffer deeply and alone because of it. The thought of telling someone, "I am suffering from depression and anxiety, and yes, it is a mental illness," is another layer of pride to swallow, another layer of acknowledging this sickness.

Each one of these milestones has its own pain, its own stress. There is no manual on what to do. There are no easy answers. And when you're in the middle of it, you are in no position to make intelligent decisions. Yet no one else can make them for you, unless you're ready to be hospitalized.

So Who is the Team?

This is why having a team of people whom you trust is so crucial. Who are these people, and what can they do for you? Here are some obvious ones:

- Go to your family doctor. Just do it, and tell him what's going on. While depression may feel like it is unique to you, it is tragically common in our over-stimulated and ridiculously busy world. Just lay it out. Have the doctor refer you to a psychiatrist for prescribing medication. Your family doctor can prescribe anti-depressants and other medications, but it is best to turn to an expert.

- Go to your pastor. If you don't have a pastor, find one quickly. I feel blessed to have the best pastor in my church, but we all should have that loyalty for the pastor who gives us the words of our dear Lord in and out of season. This pastor may be a personal friend, although I don't think that is always best. The key thing is that a pastor's pastor must be someone you trust. Tell him what's going on — the whole story, warts and all. You need to have people in your corner who are thinking clearly. There are many times even now when I am not capable of making intelligent decisions. Someone has to be able to think objectively. Ideally the pastor would be nearby, but I suppose that's not absolutely necessary.

- Talk to your wife. This may come as a shock to you, but they know what's going on. They may not be able to define it, but they know things are not right. The more your wife understands what's happening, the better off both of you will be. All she wants is for you to be well. If you're sick, she will want to help. Depression, anxiety, and other mental illnesses require a different kind of help than does a broken leg. But she loves you. Don't hide your fears from her. This is why you're married.

- Explore counseling. I'm not talking about psycho-babble. Believe me when I say I have seen psycho-babble really close up, and it is not helpful. But a good counselor can serve as a listening post, help to refine your thinking and decision making, and give you the experience of one who has helped hundreds or even thousands of patients. Most importantly, a good counselor understands exactly what you are going through. The trick is finding a counselor you trust. You might try Lutheran Social Services or other Christian counseling services in your area. Personally, I am quite leery of most generic Christian counseling. If a counselor comes from a Reformed background, he or she is going to turn you toward the Law, which is the last thing you need. If a counselor comes from the liberal wing of Christianity (if it can be called such), she or he may use a lot of Christian-sounding words, but be using a different dictionary. I am very blessed to have a solid, confessional Lutheran counselor in the LCMS. But if I didn't have such a theologically sound counselor, I would probably go to a secular counselor. (It can be easier to insert proper theology without having to first weed out wrong theology.) While pastors have a lot of unique challenges to face with mental illness, much of what they face is common.[33]

- Tell your friends what's going on. The stigma of mental illness creates this bizarre temptation to hide it from the very people that can help the most. I have a few friends in whom I confide, who have been hugely helpful. Don't be afraid; they are your friends. They'll help you if they are able, and will certainly pray for you, check in on you, and the like. Trust them.

- At some point, consider talking to key members of your congregation. This is perhaps the hardest,

---

33   You may also want to consider seeing someone who practices cognitive therapy, and not some derivation of Freudian or Jungian psychoanalysis. While every system has its flaws, cognitive therapy (or cognitive reframing) seems to have the least problems theologically. It doesn't dwell on the inherent goodness (or badness) of man, but addresses what behaviors can change in order to help your mental health.

because we super-pastors don't want our flock to know that we are weak like they are. It is arrogance that comes from a false view of the Office, and most of us succumb to it in one fashion or another. The way congregations receive this knowledge will vary, but I would start by seeking out whomever you trust the most (Notice a theme here?) and confiding in them what's happening. Discuss with them how to approach it with your parish. Because I ended up going on disability leave, I had to tell everyone. In the end it was the right decision, but it was very scary for a while. Life is like that sometimes.

This is practical, straightforward advice. But if you are suffering from depression, or know someone who is, you need to know what your real options are. A pat on the back or more sunshine is not going to cut it. You need help, and God has placed people into your life who will help you, if given the chance.

Prayer

Heavenly Father, whose mercy and compassion for Your children never fails or falters, grant me the grace and wisdom to know when I need help, whom to ask for help, and when to ask them. I don't want to ask, for I am weak and prideful. But out of your boundless love for me give me the strength to do what must be done, so that I may be healed in body and soul and continue to serve you; through Your Son, Jesus Christ, our Lord. Amen.

Points to Ponder

- Why is it so hard to tell people we love about our weaknesses?

- How would your congregation react if you told them you had a mental illness?

- How would you react if a close friend or fellow pastor told you they were going through major depression? Would you know how to help them?

Chapter Seven: The Plunge to Disability

O God, forsake me not!
Your gracious presence lend me;
Lord, lead your helpless child;
Your Holy Spirit send me
That I my course may run.
O be my light, my lot,
My staff, my rock, my shield—
O God, forsake me not![34]

It was at that point in early February that I began seriously to consider going on disability. My counselor was encouraging it. My pastor supported it. My wife thought it was the only way I would give up control and actually let go of the things that were pushing me into the ground.

I was afraid. I thought of being in a hospital or just sitting at home, staring at the wall for days at a time. I didn't want to end up like one of those mentally ill people who never recover. I didn't know how it would affect us financially. Sitting in the pew on Sunday would be torture. It was a road of uncertainty that brought only images of despair. I couldn't know then that it would save my life.

With the help of my counselor, we figured out the process under my insurance plan. All it took was a phone call. What could be harder than that?

Yet I was scared, helpless, and worried. How would my parish survive this ordeal? How much could I do for them while on disability? What about our school association? Would it wear out my fellow pastor and the school headmaster? How would this affect so many other people?

---

34   *Lutheran Service Book*, "O God, Forsake Me Not," Stanza 1 (St. Louis, MO: Concordia Publishing House, 2006), 731. Public domain.

No Option

In reality, I had no choice. I would either go on disability and focus on my own healing, or try to continue blazing away until I ended up in a hospital, or worse. I'm not sure what finally convinced me to make the call a week or two after I had all the information. It took a lot of coaxing from a lot of people to make it happen, but I finally made the call.

The transition wasn't bad. There was a two-week evaluation period during which my doctors answered questions and I filled out some paperwork (another torture). But after two weeks I was on disability. My pastor found someone to assist in my parish while I was on disability — someone I knew and trusted. It was a huge relief.

After the evaluation period I was granted partial disability, due to a clerical error on how the paperwork was filled out. My congregation, however, was wonderful. Nobody knew what to expect in all of this, and there certainly were moments of tension, but God's people took care of us. That is what matters at the end of the day. Between the generosity of our parish, other individuals, and three sister churches in our circuit, it worked financially.

How Does God Work it All Out?

One of the big fears with disability leave is finances. Most insurance plans pay disability at about 70% of your regular salary, on the understanding that because you aren't working, your expenses will be less. It doesn't make any sense to me, but that is how it works. However, we know the Lord will provide. He does, even when it seems impossible. If He condemned His own Son to death to raise you from the dead, will He not also take care of your earthly needs?

If there is a stigma hovering over mental illness, there is just as much stigma with disability leave. We think of damaged goods, less-than-ideal property, or workers that can't go 100 percent. Disability evokes sympathy and pity, as well as an attitude of condescension toward the disabled. "Thank God I am not like your other creatures…." This attitude can be directed toward anyone on disability but seems magnified in the case of mental illness. Mental illness means instability, not being able to handle things. It means never being sure what the mentally ill person can do or cannot do. It also means that the mentally ill person cannot make decisions alone. So in a sincere effort to help, sometimes people can meddle even more than is helpful.

Despite all of this, disability leave is usually a good and healthy option for those suffering from depression and anxiety. It gives you one of the things that you need the most: time free from responsibility. William Styron in his book, *Darkness Visible*, commented that it wasn't until the solace of time in the hospital that he began to find healing from his disease.[35] That solace need not happen in a hospital. It can happen at home, a friend's house, a retreat house, or many different places. But the first step is to clear your plate of everything except the absolute necessities: no responsibilities. Sleep when you want, eat when you want, be free. Structure will come in time. At the beginning, though, having that kind of absolute rest is critical in healing. Many people who go through depression manage to keep working through it and eventually get better. For the life of me I don't know how. Certainly there are different levels of illness, and they require different levels of healing.

What About Hospitalization?

I was never hospitalized for my illness. I came close on two occasions, which we will get to later. Having said that, hospitalization is not something to fear. At a hospital one is

35   William Styron, *Darkness Visible, a Memoir of Madness* (New York: Random House, 1990).

completely free of responsibilities. There is plenty of evidence that both hospitalization and outpatient care have served well over the years.[36]

By the time we got my disability figured out, I was close to hitting bottom. I foolishly didn't let go completely. I sought to keep my Sunday responsibilities and let my fellow pastor do the rest. I should have had him do everything from the start, but I thought this arrangement would disrupt the congregation the least. In fact, it made things worse, for them and for me. It forced me to put on my pastor mask one morning each week, and I ended up pouring what little energy I had into that Sunday morning task. It continued to drain me for another six weeks. It was also more difficult for the congregation, because, for many of them, Sunday morning was when they saw me. I looked fine. *What's the big problem?* It created confusion in the congregation and made things worse for me. Bad call.

The problem was not disability leave. Rather, it was one of the many foolish decisions that I made during the year I was on disability. God is merciful, though, and took care of me despite my foolishness. He used my failings for my own benefit. Only our gracious God can turn such pain into blessing.

Prayer

From God can nothing move me;
He will not step aside
But gently will reprove me
And be my constant guide.
He stretches out His hand

---

36   Cadieux, R.J. "Practical Management of Treatment-Resistant Depression," American Family Physician, December 1998; vol 58: pp 2059-62. Depression and Bipolar Support Alliance web site, "Understanding Hospitalization for Mental Health." Keller, M.B. Journal of Clinical Psychiatry, 2005; vol 66 (supp. 8): 5-12.

In evening and in morning,
My life with grace adorning
Wherever I may stand.[37]

Questions to Ponder

- What do you think of when you hear the word *disability*?

- Which holds more of a stigma for the pastor: *depression* or *disability*? Why?

- In what sense can disability status be deeply theological for your congregation and for you in the process?

---

37   Lutheran Book of Worship, "From God Can Nothing Move Me," Stanza 1 (Minneapolis, MN: Augsburg Fortress Press, 1978). Reproduced with special permission.

Chapter Eight: Forsaken

My flesh and my heart may fail
but God is the strength of my heart and my portion forever
(Ps. 73:26, ESV).

The morass of depression makes many of the things we take for granted painful, almost impossible. The physical action of getting up from bed may often be the biggest challenge of the day. Or it could be eating, getting to sleep, or talking politely with other people. Playing chase with my children became a benchmark of how I was doing. If I could play chase then it was a decent day. At one point I didn't play chase with them for a year. It was a question I heard every day. Every time my daughters asked to play chase, a knife cut my heart. But I couldn't do it; the ability just wasn't there.

Many others have written on the morass of depression far better than I. But in this chapter I want to discuss the spiritual effects of depression.

It is a very strange line to draw, no question about it. For the Christian, depression hits them at the very core of being. Can God really be doing this to me? Does He care at all? Why does He hate me so much? Am I worse than all the other sinners somehow, that I deserve this?

Because depression is an extreme turning inward upon the self, it is a fertile ground for Satan to plant his chaff of doubt and despair. He uses the fact that you have no energy, that you are trapped in the labyrinth of your own mind, to draw you away from the very things you need the most as a suffering sinner. Here are just a few.

Going to Church

How can a pastor not want to go to church? Let me count the ways. The crowds, the stimulation, the conversations, the weight of the stole upon your neck (whether you're wearing it or not), all pull you down. Perhaps more importantly though, going to the Lord's House to receive His gifts is not something pastors do well on the receiving end. I can hardly stand to listen to other people preach. It's part of the arrogance that Satan uses to attack the Office. Satan uses your own weaknesses (pride, vanity, etc.) to turn you away from the very place where you need to be the most. For me, it was unbelievable torture to sit in the pew with my family. In my mind, it was *more* work than being in the chancel. I had kids crawling over me, people talking around me when they should have been listening, and the underlying feeling that I was simply in the *wrong place*. I don't belong in the nave. I belong in the pulpit. So while I was more or less there every week, whether I was in the chancel or not it was utterly draining. It would take me several days to recover.

I remember quite distinctly the day that my son, Richard, was baptized. I had been on disability for about seven weeks. I actually wrote a sermon for the occasion. It was getting harder and harder to do. We had a house full of relatives. It is one of the great joys of being a pastor. But I felt nothing. My illness had robbed me even of the joy of my son's entrance into God's kingdom through Holy Baptism. Fortunately, feelings do not make a Baptism valid or invalid. God was at work that day, and continues to work in Richard even now.

Individual Confession and Absolution

We haven't talked much about the need to have a trusted pastor to take care of you. Frankly it is a tragedy of our day that most pastors don't have a pastor for themselves. Personally, I believe this is one of the big contributing causes to pastoral attrition. Where this really has an impact is in individual confession and absolution. No matter how good a counselor you have, a counselor is not a pastor. Don't expect him (or her) to be a pastor, and don't expect your pastor to be a counselor. Your pastor is there to forgive your sins, bring you the healing balm of the Gospel, and carry you in prayer when you can't pray for yourself (more on this in a minute). This is most clear in confession and absolution. There can be no question what you are there for, namely to hear and receive the Gospel.

Yet it is the Source of this Gospel that keeps the suffering pastor away. I was angry with God. When I had the energy to think straight, when I felt anything at all, I was simply angry. I didn't want to talk to God or hear from Him. I didn't have the energy to put into another "relationship". So your pastor has to seek you out, pray for you whether you want it or not, and treat you almost like a shut-in. This is what you need, even if it feels unnatural and weird.

Prayer with God

Prayer disappeared for me. Praying the daily office (which we did regularly at our school) was impossible. I couldn't do it; I couldn't preach to 25 little Lutherans and their teachers. I could barely even be there. The words meant absolutely nothing to me. This was true both for daily prayer at school and personal prayer at home. It simply vanished. Why?

I think the reason again is similar to confession and absolution. I didn't want to talk to God. If God wouldn't just fix things now, and in my way, then He was of no use to me. I didn't have the energy to plead with Him. The persistence of the Canaanite woman or the blind beggar was not mine. That required an active faith, which I didn't have. All I could do was stare and suffer.

I went months without praying. I said the words at church, but they simply rolled off my tongue and meant nothing. This aspect of depression was perhaps the most painful for me; it left me abandoned and alone, bereft of God and man alike — at least in my mind. This was as close as I got to prayer:

My God, my God, why have you forsaken me?

Why are you so far from saving me, from the words of my groaning? (Ps. 22:1, ESV)

So where is hope to be found when all of our Lord's sources of hope and healing either disappear or leave you feeling worse off than you were before? That is the sickness of this disease. It robs you of everything you love, and insulates you so tightly that it is almost impossible for anyone who loves you to get in.

This is the crucible of the theology of the cross, right there. The cross is painful. It is bitter and cruel. The abandonment of God and man is the most painful experience that anyone can go through. It cannot be academically dissected, though many have tried, to varying degrees of success.[38]

For a time, these very things that our Lord uses to create and sustain faith happened without feeling — sometimes less frequently, and sometimes not at all (especially in the case of prayer). Yet this is where our Lord uses His gifts to the greatest benefit. We so easily forget that faith is a gift of God (Eph. 2:8-9) and not an act of will on our part.

Faith does not exist on the basis of an illness or lack thereof. Faith does not survive because we try harder, feel more, or think more about God. Faith and trust come solely by God's gracious work through His Son, Jesus Christ. God uses His means of salvation to create and sustain faith. His Word, Baptism, Absolution, and Holy Communion are His tools for keeping us in the one true faith.

---

38   Some of the more recent and more successful approaches to this include C.S. Lewis' classic work, *The Problem of Pain*, and to a lesser extent, *A Grief Observed*. Lutheran treatments include Gregory Schulz, *The Problem of Suffering: A Father's Thoughts on the Suffering, Death, and Life of His Children* (Milwaukee, WI: Northwestern Publishing House, 1996), and Gerhard Forde, *On Being a Theologian of the Cross* (Grand Rapids, MI: William B. Eerdmans, 1997).

What Does This Mean?

So what does this mean for the sufferer? There are dark times when you are alone, when you have been abandoned by all, when your very mind and body are screaming at you like Jobs friends, "Curse God and die!" (Job 2:9). It is precisely at these moments, when everything else has been stripped away, that the promises of God are the only thing that will sustain you. They will sustain you, whether you feel like they will or not, whether you feel you can pray or not, even if going to church seems empty and flat. God will never abandon you.

This is the paradox. Your mind and body, maybe even your friends and family, may tell you (like Job's friends), that you are alone. But you are never alone. Remember St. Paul's glorious words:

> Likewise the Spirit helps us in our weakness. For we do not know what to pray for as we ought, but the Spirit himself intercedes for us with groanings too deep for words. And he who searches hearts knows what is the mind of the Spirit, because the Spirit intercedes for the saints according to the will of God. And we know that for those who love God all things work together for good, for those who are called according to his purpose. For those whom he foreknew he also predestined to be conformed to the image of his Son, in order that he might be the firstborn among many brothers. And those whom he predestined he also called, and those whom he called he also justified, and those whom he justified he also glorified (Rom. 8:26-30, ESV).

These are not just words. God's Word does what it says. When you can't "inwardly digest" the Word as you wish, it still does what our Lord promises. When confession is lost upon your lips, our Lord forgives your sins out of His mercy, for He will not let a sickness or weakness on your part deny you what you truly need, namely His healing Word of forgiveness. And when prayer is something that you *used* to do, the Spirit prays with you and for you, in ways that we cannot even fathom. This is the mercy of God. He does not abandon you, period. You are His child, His son, and nothing can change that.

Prayer

Sin, disturb my soul no longer:
 I am baptized into Christ!
I have comfort even stronger:
 Jesus' cleansing sacrifice.
Should a guilty conscience seize me
Since my Baptism did release me
 In a dear forgiving flood,
 Sprinkling me with Jesus' blood?[39]

Questions to Ponder

- Why would a pastor, or any Christian, lose sight of the basic foundations of the Christian faith?

- Is it possible for an illness to make receiving the gifts of God more difficult?

- How does God work for you and in you when it seems as though there is nothing there?

---

39   Robert Voelker, "God's Own Child, I Gladly Say It," Stanza 2. Used with permission.

Chapter Nine: Thinking the Unthinkable

What God ordains is always good:
Though I the cup am drinking
   Which savors now of bitterness,
   I take it without shrinking.
      For after grief
      God gives relief,
My heart with comfort filling
And all my sorrow stilling.[40]

I thought as I was going through the changes in medication, figuring out disability, fighting my own personal demons, and trying to learn how to give up control, that I had reached the bottom. I could go no lower. I was wrong.

As I got ready for the day's events on Good Friday (two months into disability), my grip on reality was fragile, but holding. I could function most days for a few hours, as long as I poured everything I had into that time. Writing sermons had stopped months before. Making calls was gone; I couldn't take the people. Greeting people after church was torture. Yet somehow I had come to believe that I could still get through all of this, keep working, be a husband and father, and hang together. Then the phone rang.

"Hello! This is your representative from Broadspire, Incorporated. Is this Mr. Peperkorn?" The voice was drearily cheerful.

"This is me," I replied.

"I'm calling to inform you that our independent review board has determined that you are no longer qualified for disability, effective April first" (two weeks before.) Her tone was matter of fact, just one more call to check off the list of

---

40   *Lutheran Service Book*, "What God Ordains Is Always Good," Stanza 5 (St. Louis, MO: Concordia Publishing House, 2006), 760. Public domain.

activities.

"How is that possible?" I asked. "Did my doctors recommend this? What happened?"

"There is an appeal process which you may choose to undertake if you believe this determination was in error. Would you like to know the process?" The speech was ready and expected. She knew the script.

I was numb. I mumbled some response and hung up the phone. My wife asked what had happened. I think I told her. I sat and stared at the computer for what seemed like a lifetime. My future was draining out of me like blood from a cut artery. There was nothing I could do. This was beyond my control.

There was no way I could get better if I had to work full-time. I wasn't really getting better even working part-time. The thought of the yoke of the pastoral office being thrust upon me again, against my will, loomed before me.

I slept. I stared at the wall. Somehow I got up. I called my therapist and left a message. Like a walking dead man I moved about our house, oblivious to my wife, our young children, the telephone, everything. What I was searching for I couldn't find. I needed hope, a future, a reason to live. I couldn't see past my own misery and pain. I wanted it gone — really gone. I couldn't wait for some magical drug or therapeutic insight to flip the switch and make things right. The darkness had taken me. It was only a matter of time.

The thought of my own death had only held a theoretical appeal up to that point. Most people think about suicide at some point in their life, perhaps even often. In moments of sadness or hardship, times in life that seem extremely difficult or trying, a way out is very appealing. We would be lying to ourselves if we said it never crossed our minds. But it's just a fleeting thought.

This was different. For the clinically depressed, suicide is a 900-pound gorilla in the room. It's your constant companion, ever in the shadows. As the light and darkness become just darkness, suicide steps forward, enticing, innocent, the way out that can solve all your problems. My thoughts moved from the theoretical to the how and when phase. If I couldn't stay on disability, I couldn't get better. I was no use to anyone alive, and I was a huge burden on my wife and family. Why bother any longer? Just get it over with and trust that God will understand. Just figure out how to do it.

Being on part-time disability meant, obviously, that despite these raging thoughts in my head, I still had a job to do somehow. So I put on the uniform (an increasingly painful process), and went to our sister church to assist with the Tre Ore service. I wasn't preaching, just assisting with readings and the liturgy. I don't remember when I told the pastor (who was also my father confessor) what had happened; it was probably before the service, which was a blur. It's a wonder I got through it at all, doing readings, following the liturgy, etc. These things come pretty naturally to me; I must have functioned on auto-pilot.

Hearing my own pastor's meditation on the death of Christ was a gift. He put the proverbial silver bullet into my enemy, which brought me some small amount of comfort. But sometimes a small amount goes a really long way.

After the service, we went out for coffee. He listened, just sitting with me through my quiet mourning over my life. He wouldn't let me go until he knew I was safe. Whether he realizes it or not, he saved my life. Without his "I'm not going away" presence, I don't know what I would have done. It would not have been good, that's for sure. But he listened with utmost patience, and then talked me out of the pit enough for me to go home and rest. It was a very good thing.

I went home and slept. I watched a movie on my computer. Then I had to get ready for our own Good Friday service that evening. I would be preaching at that service. Fortunately the sermon was done, albeit a rerun. I had another pastor assisting me, which was very good. The service went fine, though I don't remember it. I do remember preaching about how Jesus' death brings life to all. And I remember the irony of contemplating my own death on the day we commemorate our Lord's death in our behalf.

The day ended, and I came out alive. It was not my efforts, but the people God had put in my path who kept me here. On my own, I would surely have been lost. But I was not lost, because I was never alone, even though the demons in my mind were telling me I was.

That was the low point for me. It was the day that convinced me that without real rest, real quiet, and lack of responsibility I would never get better. That realization was one of the chief steps toward healing for me. I didn't know whether that rest should be in a hospital, at someone's house, or elsewhere. But the fact that I needed it became very apparent.

The Christian and Suicide

Could this happen to you? Believe it. Anyone is susceptible to events like mine. Satan revels in them. As with Saul, Judas, and so many others, Satan can use any external force to drive us to despair. Martin Luther once wrote:

Since the devil is not only a liar, but also a murderer [John 8:44], he constantly seeks our life. He wreaks his vengeance whenever he can afflict our bodies with misfortune and harm. Therefore, it happens that he often breaks men's necks or drives them to insanity, drowns some, and moves many to commit suicide and to many other terrible disasters [e.g., Mark 9:17–22].[41]

---

41   Paul Timothy McCain, (ed.), *Concordia: The Lutheran Confessions – A Reader's Edition of the Book of Concord*, 2nd ed. (St. Louis, MO: Concordia Publishing House, 2007), 422. Used with permission.

This is so true, and a disease of the mind is the perfect ground for Satan to plant his sick weeks of unbelief.

Is it a sin to consider such thoughts as suicide? This is one of the many questions of guilt that trouble the clinically depressed. Self-death is a sin, but it is only a sin. Jesus died for all our sins, even suicide or worse. We are often placed in impossible situations, where we sin if we do, and sin if we don't. Even if external forces (extended illness, loss of work, etc.) put us in such a situation, sin is still sin. But more importantly, Jesus' forgiveness is still forgiveness.

Christ came to take our death. We really died in the font, not when our body is laid to rest. This means that no matter what terrible thoughts you harbor in your soul, in the midst of your despair, Christ is there. You may not be able to see Him, feel Him, or touch Him, but He is there. You are washed in Baptism; you are cleansed in His name. You are His holy child, beloved in His sight. Yes, you suffer. It is painful. But suffer as the redeemed. For you will come out whole and undefiled in the end.

Prayer

O eternal and merciful God, I give eternal thanks to You that so far You have guarded me from countless evils and provided me with the protection of Your holy angels. Your gracious acts by which You have protected me from evil are even more numerous than the acts by which You give good things to me. Whenever I see others suffer evils of body and soul, I acknowledge Your kind mercy toward me. If, indeed, I am free from such cares and evils, I owe this only to Your goodness.

How great is the power of the devil. How great is his deceitfulness. Every time that wicked spirit, our powerfully cunning enemy, has tried to condemn me,

I have been able to flee his net and find safety behind the shield of Your kindness and the protection of the angels. Can anyone count the traps of the devil? Who can count the times You have protected us from his traps? When I sleep, Your providential eye watches over me to prevent that hellish enemy, who walks around like a roaring lion (I Peter 5:8), from surprising me with his traps and powers. When Satan attacks me with his temptations by day, the strength of Your right hand comforts me in the kindest way and prevents that deceitful tempter from enticing me into his snares. When a countless army of evils threatens me, the camps of Your angels (Psalm 34:7) surround me like a wall of fire (Zechariah 2:5).

Even the most trifling and insignificant creature threatens me with various dangers. How great and boundless is Your kindness that You keep me safe from them. My soul and body are inclined to fall into sin. Because this is so, kindest Father, You rule my soul by Your Spirit, my body by an angelic shield. You command Your angels to guard me wherever I go and to support me with their hands so my feet are not dashed against a stone (Psalm 91:11-12). Because of Your mercy, I am not destroyed. New dangers surround me every day, therefore Your mercies are new to me every morning (Lamentations 3:22-23). You do not slumber or sleep, O faithful and watchful Keeper of soul and body (Psalm 121:4). Your grace is the shade at my right hand that keeps the scorching midday rays of open and harsh persecution from striking me down and guards me from the calamities and hidden ambushes of the night (Psalms 121:6). You watch over my coming in, direct my going forth, and govern my going out (Psalm 121:8). For this kindness, I will sing praise eternally to You and to Your name. Amen.[42]

Questions to Ponder

- Is suicide always a sin? Why or why not?
- What do you do when you are thinking of hurting yourself or others, for whatever reason?
- How do you know that Christ is with you even in those darkest moments?

---

42   Johann Gerhard, *Meditations on Divine Mercy: A Classic Treasury of Devotional Prayers*, trans. Matthew Harrison (St. Louis, MO: Concordia Publishing House, 2003), 88-89.

Chapter 10: The Rest I Needed

But those who wait on the LORD shall renew their strength; they shall mount up with wings like eagles, they shall run and not be weary, they shall walk and not faint (Is. 40:31, NKJV).

Come to Me, all you who labor and are heavy laden, and I will give you rest (Matt.11:28, NKJV).

After Good Friday it was very obvious to me, my counselor, my wife, my pastor, and pretty much everyone who knew the story that I needed a change. We discussed options. There basically were three: go to a "mental health care" hospital; enter an outpatient program; or stay for a couple weeks with someone who had a very quiet and peaceful house. Any one of the three were good options, although I was obviously not excited about the first two.

I ended up staying with some friends whose home was near the seminary where I had studied and worked for years. Their children were grown, and they were both very engaged people. Their house was quiet. I could attend chapel if I wanted. I could sleep in, watch TV or movies, or read. I could play golf. I had absolutely nothing I needed to do for two weeks. It was bliss.

What made this time so critical for my healing was the complete absence of responsibility. Responsibility weighs down the depressed person in ways that few can understand. The parish, my family, the insurance fiasco, the related financial trials, my own desire to control my life had pushed me down to the point where I couldn't even look up for fear of being crushed.

A time of freedom was liberating. It enabled me to step back from all of these events, simply not think of them for a while, and then turn around and view them with new eyes.

We are so seldom given the opportunity to do this, and it is such a shame.

This is where the Roman Catholic Church has historically done much better than Lutherans in terms of caring for their priests. They have retreat centers all over the country. Certainly some of their theology makes the healing flawed, but the concept of a place of quiet and rest is a good, healthy, and even biblical concept. Jesus often went by Himself to pray alone (Matthew 11), and the Psalms often speak of solitude and quiet with God.

As I look back on the experience and how it shaped my healing in terms of time, medication, therapy, and the medicine of the soul, this was the new beginning for me. It took that level of complete disengagement for me to be able to start over.

There were setbacks along the way. The insurance fiasco continued for a couple more months. The personal financial troubles related to it will take years to work themselves out. The wear and tear on my parish was very tough, as it also was on my family, my pastor, and everyone else involved in my healing. Some months later things got so bad again that I had to take another retreat for a couple weeks, to a different family's home. But the effect was the same. It gave me simplicity, peace, community if I wanted it, and friends who cared for me without making demands.

After a long, long journey, I began to see things a little more clearly. There was less fog, more sunshine. I began to catch glimpses of joy. I could enjoy a few moments with my children just being happy, without measuring how much I could take before I had to leave. I did a sermon, written from scratch, here or there. The Word of God, slowly took root in new places in my soul, places I never knew existed. Prayer began to trickle, then flow into a little creek. But it came.

I wouldn't say that I am healed. I know my limitations, and I know that things are not back to normal. Maybe they will never be the same again. Maybe they will be better, different, less focused on the tasks at hand and more focused on the gifts that only God can bring through the Holy Spirit in the Word. But I can preach again. I can hear my people's sins and forgive them in Jesus' name. I can pray the liturgy with my people and know that this is who I am again. The excruciating pain of depression cost me much. In the end, though, this suffering has strengthened me. I could never see it at the time, but it is nonetheless true. Suffering is a sign of the love of God upon your life. It is a gift, not a curse.

There is peace. There is hope. There is a future. These things are always there in Christ, no matter how dark the road may be. Just because you cannot feel, taste, touch, or even hear Him, these promises of God are no less true. His Word is powerful and effective, even if it feels like dead words upon your heart. The promises given in your Baptism do not fade away and disappear because you are in despair and darkness. That is *exactly* when your Baptism may be all that is holding you together. Perhaps Martin Luther said it best:

> In this way one sees what a great, excellent thing Baptism is. It delivers us from the devil's jaws and makes us God's own. It suppresses and takes away sin and then daily strengthens the new man. It is working and always continues working until we pass from this estate of misery to eternal glory.[43]

If this is true of Baptism, this is also true of God's great means of the Spirit, the Lord's Supper. For remember, "he who is worthy and well prepared has faith in these words, given and shed for you."[44] Notice what it doesn't say. It doesn't say "who

---

43   Paul Timothy McCain, (ed.), *Concordia: The Lutheran Confessions – A Reader's Edition of the Book of Concord*, 2nd ed. (St. Louis, MO: Concordia Publishing House, 2007), 431. Used with permission.

44   *Lutheran Service Book*, (St. Louis, MO: Concordia Publishing House, 2006), 327.

feels forgiven" or "who is happy and joyful after receiving communion" or "who has a strong and powerful faith that everyone looks up to and admires". Do not be afraid. Our Lord said that faith the size of a mustard seed could move mountains (Matt. 17:20). Remember, though, that faith is a gift from God, not your own doing (Eph. 2:8-9). Depression cannot steal your faith from you. It cannot rob you of the promises that God has inscribed with the blood of His own Son. There is a light in the darkness. It will not fade away.

Prayer

Almighty and most merciful God, in this earthly life we endure sufferings and death before we enter into eternal glory. Grant us grace at all times to subject ourselves to Your holy will and to continue steadfast in the true faith to the end of our lives that we may know the peace and joy of the blessed hope of the resurrection of the dead and of the glory of the world to come; through Jesus Christ, our Lord. Amen.[45]

Questions to Ponder

* Why is it that rest and freedom from responsibility can help with healing?

* Where does our Lord and His suffering on the cross fit into our understanding of suffering?

* What is the future we all have in Christ, the Suffering One?

---

45 *Lutheran Service Book*, (St. Louis, MO: Concordia Publishing House, 2006), 317. Used with permission.

Epilogue

O God, O Lord of heav'n and earth,
Thy living finger never wrote
That life should be an aimless mote,
A deathward drift from futile birth.
They Word meant life triumphant hurled
In splendor through Thy broken world.
Since light awoke and life began,
Thou has desired Thy life for man.[46]

There is no magic bullet when it comes to depression. The causes are varied, the treatments are varied, and the recovery is varied. I write this only a little more than a year since I went on disability, and I am just now getting back into the rhythm of parish life.

The key thing is that I *am* getting back into the rhythm of parish life. There can be an end to depression. Or perhaps more accurately, you can come to understand depression as a part of you. I don't mean in some sort of hospice sense that death is natural or anything like that. Suffering changes you, whether it is depression, death, persecution, or another form. It does change you. You may receive this change as a gift from our Lord who loves you and seeks to draw you closer to Him. Or you may look at it as a curse and a sign that God doesn't really care. Suffering always creates in us a longing to be free of this earthly life and to join our Lord forever in heaven. This is good. It helps us to understand that this life is transitory, but the Word of the Lord endures forever.

Suffering can also provide the powerful reality of an insight, a little tiny glimpse into the suffering of our Lord on the cross. Because of that glimpse, the suffering pastor also

---

46 *O God, O Lord of Heaven and Earth*, Stanza 1 (Minneapolis, MN: Augsburg Fortress Press, 1994). Reproduced with special permission.

has a glimpse into the lives of his people and the suffering they endure — big and little, important or seemingly trivial.

I am a better pastor because of depression. God has chastened me, taught me the hard lesson of humility, and given me some small insight into the pain and trials that my people deal with every day. It is a gift, even if the suffering itself is a result of our fallen and sinful world.

Reentry into the parish is not easy. My counselor tells me that it is four times easier to take a call to a new parish than to try to start over at your current parish. Most of the things that were difficult before are still difficult for me (making calls in particular). There are times when I look at the week and wonder how I will make it. But those times are slowly happening less and less.

It's also hard to restrain myself from falling into the same "super pastor" habits that contributed to my problems in the first place. Numerous people continue to remind me to slow down and not take on new things. They usually get through to me.

So I continue to serve where God has placed me, and wait upon Him for what the future will bring. Nonetheless, as a pastor it is not as if you have control over such things. If you are called elsewhere, you consider it. If not, then you work in the vineyard where the Lord has placed you.

Coming back to the vineyard may be difficult. Your parishioners may be used to you not being there, or at least not being there in the way they would want or expect. They may even have to relearn what it means to have a pastor. But you can teach them. You have been down the dark road. With patience and endurance, you can give them what you did not have to give before.

I have found that I listen more and talk less. It's hard to believe from a talker like me. But I know that when you are suffering, you need to share that suffering so that you do not suffer alone. A pastor can share in that suffering with his flock. A pastor actually suffers with his flock, just as our Lord suffers with us — through every heartache, every temptation, every trial of body and soul that we face.

Getting back into the rhythm is hard, sometimes very hard. I tire easily. It is still common for me to receive too much stimulation and just shut down. I have to plan out every day and gauge what I can handle on that day. It is a daily learning process. But by the mercy of God, given through his Word and Holy Sacraments, each day begins anew. Some are better than others, but they are all days lived in His time and in His way.

Be patient with yourself. Don't expect life to go back to normal. Things will be different for you, your family, and your parish. At the end of the day I believe they will be better, because you have gained wisdom through your suffering, and wisdom cannot have a price put on it. Let things flow as they will for a time. Simply focus on what it means to be a pastor, and let the rest go. You may find, in the end, that some things that seemed crucial were never that important.

God can and will use you as His holy instrument, giving out His gifts to His people. He will see you through this, just as He has been faithful to countless generations before you. Don't be afraid. Christ is with you on the dark road.

Prayer

Lord Jesus Christ, with us abide,
For round us falls the eventide.
O let your Word, that saving light,
Shine forth undimmed into the night.[47]

---

47 *Lutheran Service Book*, "Lord Jesus Christ, with Us Abide," Text, (sts 1.) (St. Louis, MO: Concordia Publishing House, 1982), LSB 585. Used with permission.

Questions to Ponder

- What makes reentry into the parish ministry so difficult?
- What is the greatest temptation when returning to full-time ministry?
- How have you changed through this experience?

Appendix I: What to Do if a Loved One Suffers from Depression

One of the most difficult things to figure out is how to help someone in need. If someone has a broken leg, you know what to do: Call the doctor! But what if they are mentally ill, whether it is depression, anxiety, or some other illness? Here are a few suggestions to help get you started:

Pray

Someone who is suffering from depression is isolated by their mind. They can't handle contact with other people. It is almost physically painful to interact. By praying for them you are connecting them to God and the communion of saints, which is what they need more than anything else. Pray for them, because they may not be able to pray for themselves.

Talk to Them

Despite how difficult it is to interact with other people, the clinically depressed need interaction. Keep it short and to the point. Give a smile, a hug, a friendly word that you know things are hard for them and that you are praying for them. These things can make the difference between a dark and dreary day, and one where the light of God's love starts to shine through.

Talk to their Spouse

In all likelihood their spouse is suffering as much or more than the ill person. Take them out for a cup of coffee. Listen. Pray for them and with them. Be a sympathetic ear and offer to help. Sometimes offering to watch the kids for a couple of hours can give the suffering spouse a much-needed break from feeling like a single parent. The little things do matter.

Give Them Space, but Don't Avoid Them

Because personal interaction is so difficult and painful, the clinically depressed need space. Don't expect much from them. Don't avoid them, but give them room to heal. Use a gesture of kindness you know they would appreciate. Let them know you are are thinking of them and praying for them, but don't become one more thing for them to feel guilty about.

Don't Give Up

This is certainly the hardest. Don't give up! They need you. You may be their lifeline to the faith that can sustain them through their dark hours. It may require great persistence on your part, but don't grow weary of doing good. It will be to their great benefit and your joy.

Appendix II: Recommended Reading

On Depression

Greene-McCreight, Kathryn. *Darkness is My Only Companion: A Christian Response to Mental Illness*. Grand Rapids: Brazos Press, 2006.

Karp, David A. *Speaking of Sadness: Depression, Disconnection, and the Meanings of Illness*. Oxford University Press, USA, 1997.

On Anxiety

Burke, William. *Protect Us From All Anxiety: Meditations for the Depressed (Solace for Survivors)*. Chicago: ACTA Publications, 1999.

For the Families of Loved Ones

Karp, David A. *The Burden of Sympathy: How Families Cope With Mental Illness*. New York: Oxford University Press, USA, 2002.

On the Theology of the Cross

Forde, Gerhard O., and Martin Luther. *On Being a Theologian of the Cross: Reflections on Luther's Heidelberg Disputation, 1518 (Theology)*. Grand Rapids: Wm. B. Eerdmans Publishing Company, 1997.

On Pastoral Burnout

Hoge, Dean R., and Jacqueline E. Wenger. *Pastors in Transition: Why Clergy Leave Local Church Ministry (Pulpit and Pew Series)*. Grand Rapids: Wm. B. Eerdmans Publishing Company, 2005.

Preus, Robert D. "Clergy Mental Health and the Doctrine of Justification." *Concordia Theological Quarterly* 48, no. 2 & 3 (1984): 113-23.

Prayers and other Devotional Works

Deffner, Donald L. *Prayers for People Under Pressure.* Milwaukee: Northwestern Publishing House, 1992.

Gerhard, Johann. *Meditations on Divine Mercy: A Classic Treasury of Devotional Prayers.* Concordia Publishing House, 2003.

Kinnamon, Scot, ed. *Treasury of Daily Prayer.* St. Louis: Concordia Publishing House, 2008.

Lutheran Book of Prayer. Rev. ed. Saint Louis: Concordia Publishing House, 2005.

Lutheran Service Book. St. Louis: Concoria Publishing House, 2006.

Addendum

By Dr. Harold L. Senkbeil

No matter if you are a pastor or a lay person, Rev. Peperkorn's repeated reference to "my pastor" may have caught you off guard. Most of us who sit in the pews Sunday after Sunday view our pastors as in a class by themselves — a notch or two above us, most certainly — and invulnerable, spiritually speaking. Why ever would they need a pastor? They *are* pastors. They pretty much know all there is to know about God; they have a seminary diploma and the credentials to prove it. Week after week they are busy with God and the things of God. It seems incredible that they should need anyone to minister to them, since they are constantly ministering to us so effectively.

But that's just the problem. When a man is constantly giving out to others without ever taking anything in, he soon runs out of things to give. He runs dry. He becomes depleted, both spiritually and emotionally. The problem is, his congregation has a contractual right to keep on receiving his ministry even after he has nothing left. That's a recipe for burnout. It leads to perfunctory, mechanical performance in the ministry. Worst of all, it exacerbates the kind of mental numbness and emotional darkness that Pastor Peperkorn has so candidly laid bare for our inspection.

If you're a pastor, there's a pretty strong likelihood that you too were surprised by Todd's "my pastor" references — but for different reasons. Unlike many parishioners, you know that you are in no special class spiritually speaking. Like all your members, you're only human. Not only do you put your pants on one leg at a time just as they do, but you share the same sinful nature as every sheep and lamb in the flock you care for. So it's not being some sort of spiritual superman that sets you apart — what is it, then?

True enough, you have been set apart. That's what call and ordination is all about: a man, actually quite an ordinary man by all other standards, is consecrated for ministry and given an extraordinary responsibility. He is placed by God Himself into an office that Jesus expressly designed for the benefit and welfare of His beloved bride, the church.

But God never intended His ministers to be lone rangers. Christ, after all, sent His disciples out in teams, two by two. The apostles took pains to see that their ministry remained collegial. Why is it, then that modern pastors live such solitary lives spiritually speaking? I don't claim to have the complete answer to this dilemma, but I'm wondering if a big part of the problem is that we pastors have been our own worst enemies in this department. We have made our divine calling into a human profession. We have become practitioners in a profession, rather than servants in a craft. And over the years, our profession has gradually morphed into a business; a godly business, to be sure, but a business nonetheless. A lot of pastors complain about commercialization and salesmanship in the church, but let's face it — we've all had a hand in it. Slowly but surely we've come to believe that our personal ingenuity and creativity is more important than what the Holy Spirit has given us to do by means of His Word and Sacrament.

We've become entrepreneurs, in other words. And entrepreneurs are automatically competitors, not allies. No wonder, then, that the modern ministry is such a lonely profession. No wonder that we find ourselves often isolated and frequently depleted. Who wants to turn to a competitor for help, after all? And so we struggle bravely on. But we struggle alone; and that's not good.

Dietrich Bonhoeffer wrote that there is no man more alone than a man who is alone with his sin. When we're left alone in our sin, we're sitting ducks for the devil. That old ancient foe ceaselessly seeks to destroy God's church. It's no wonder that the pastor (and his family) bear the brunt of his attack; for if he can derail the pastor's ministry he can sabotage the work of the Holy Spirit.

You may remember that it was Rev. Peperkorn's pastor who kept vigil with him that dark Good Friday when suicide loomed large. That pastor saved his life, he reports. And how did he do it? He simply listened; he mourned with him, he was a "'I'm not going away' presence." Friends do that, of course. But this pastor was more than a friend; he served as the shepherd of Todd's soul. He regularly heard his confession, he repeatedly visited him and his family in their deepest need, he spoke God's Word to console them, he prayed with them and for them.

No matter where we are on the spectrum of mental and emotional health, we all need such a pastor. We need someone with whom we may share our boldest dreams, our fondest hopes, our honest fears, our abysmal failures. We need someone before whom we can confess our sins and from whose mouth we can hear the objective Word of the Gospel absolution, someone who will pray for us and with us and then bless us in the strong and abiding Name of the Holy Trinity.

It's unethical, you know, for physicians to prescribe their own medication; yet many — perhaps most — pastors self-medicate with God's Word. No one patronizes a barber with shaggy hair or seeks dental care from a dentist with no teeth. Sure, every pastor must tend his own soul as well as those of the entire flock where God has placed him as spiritual overseer. But we are not made to go solo in the ministry; every shepherd needs to be shepherded as well.

But where to look? How does a pastor find a pastor for himself? Allow me to suggest a few parameters I've discovered over the years:

1. Don't ask a buddy in the ministry. While we definitely need to cultivate friendships among

colleagues, it's best to keep these vocations distinct. When the same man serves you as friend and as pastor, one or the other role will usually suffer.

2. Don't enter into a reciprocal shepherding relationship with a fellow pastor. While we should definitely bear one another's burdens in the church, the clear demarcations of serving as either pastor or penitent are crucial in retaining the clarity and objectivity of the ministry of God's Word.

3. Don't worry that you will appear weak in the eyes of your peers. We're allies, not competitors, remember? If we believe the Word we preach and the Sacraments we administer are for the actual forgiveness, life, and salvation of God's people, we will be honored when a brother pastor comes to us seeking those same gifts.

4. Do seek pastoral help from a colleague in the ministry who demonstrates that he honors the office he holds by the respect and love he has for the Good Shepherd and the sheep and lambs of his flock (even those he finds hard to get along with).

But don't go it alone. I'm reminded of an old cops 'n robbers TV show. Every episode was introduced by a briefing for the police officers from their precinct captain. His closing warning was always the same: "…and remember, it's dangerous out there." The diligent pastor must also be vigilant about his own spiritual safety as he daily contends against devil, world, and — often trickiest of all — his own sinful flesh. Thank God, you're no lone ranger in the work you've been given to do. You have a champion who fights for you: Jesus Christ, the Righteous One. And He has promised to serve you in the ministry of your brother.

—